LOW CHOLESTEROL FOOD LIST AND COOKBOOK

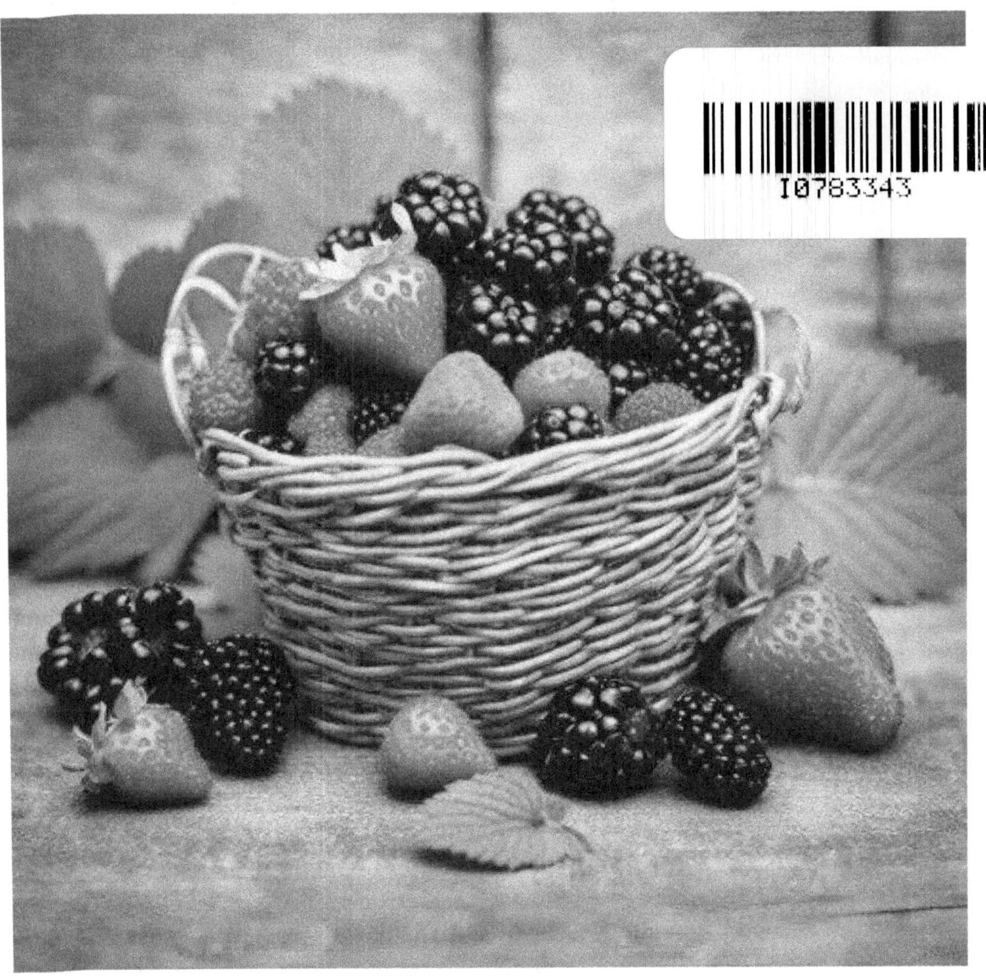

Natalie Pina

DISCLAIMER

The content within this book reflects my thoughts, experiences, and beliefs. It is meant for informational and entertainment purposes. While I have taken great care to provide accurate information, I cannot guarantee the absolute correctness or applicability of the content to every individual or situation. Please consult with relevant professionals for advice specific to your needs.

Contact the Author

Thank you for reading my book! I would love to hear from you, whether you have feedback, questions, or just want to share your thoughts. Your feedback means a lot to me and helps me improve as a writer.

Please don't hesitate to reach out to me through

drnataliepina@gmail.com

I look forward to connecting with my readers and appreciate your support in this literary journey. Your thoughts and comments are valuable to me.

<u>ABOUT THE AUTHOR</u>

Welcome to the rich tapestry of my life, where the blending of medicine and culinary arts has shaped my journey. I am Dr. Natalie Pina, a devoted healer, loving mother, and culinary enthusiast. Join me as I unravel the intricate Flavors of health and wellness, weaving together personal anecdotes, professional triumphs, and the transformative power of food.

My journey into the world of healing cuisine began in the heart of my grandmother's kitchen. Surrounded by the aromas of simmering spices and bubbling pots, I learned the profound connection between food and well-being. These early experiences ignited a flame within me, propelling me toward a career where medicine and gastronomy intersect.

As I navigated the demanding terrain of medical training, I encountered my own health challenges. Struggling with nutrient deficiencies, I faced a pivotal moment of realization: the healer needed healing. This personal journey of self-discovery fuelled my passion for nutrition and drove me to explore innovative approaches to holistic wellness.

Armed with a newfound appreciation for the healing power of food, I embarked on a mission to bridge the gap between medicine and culinary arts. As both a physician and a part-time chef, I witnessed the profound impact of nourishing cuisine on my patients' lives. Through tailored meal plans, cooking workshops, and culinary prescriptions, I empowered individuals to take control of their health one delicious bite at a time.

Driven by my love for cooking and healing, I embarked on a journey of culinary innovation. From my kitchen laboratory emerged a plethora of nutrient-rich creations, each one a testament to my commitment to flavor and nourishment. Whether crafting gluten-free delicacies or vitamin-enriched delights, I endeavored to make healthy eating a joyous and satisfying experience for all.

As I reflect on my life's work, I am filled with gratitude for the countless lives touched by my passion for healing cuisine. From patients overcoming chronic conditions to families embracing vibrant health, each success story reaffirms the transformative potential of food as medicine. As I continue to advocate for wellness and culinary creativity, I am reminded that the true essence of healing lies in the joy of nourishing both body and soul.

<u>HOW TO THIS COOKBOOK</u>

Using a food list cookbook can simplify your meal planning and grocery shopping while expanding your culinary repertoire. Here's how to make the most of it:

1. **Familiarize Yourself**: Start by flipping through the cookbook to get an overview of the recipes and ingredients. Take note of any sections or chapters that catch your interest.

2. **Select Recipes**: Browse through the recipes and choose the ones you want to try. Consider factors such as cooking time, complexity, and availability of ingredients.

3. **Check the Food Lists**: Most food list cookbooks categorize ingredients by type, such as proteins, grains, vegetables, and spices. Locate the food lists corresponding to your chosen recipes.

4. **Make a Shopping List**: Referencing the ingredients listed for each recipe, jot down the items you need to buy. Organize your list according to the categories provided in the cookbook to streamline your shopping experience.

5. **Grocery Shopping**: Armed with your list, head to the grocery store or market. As you shop, cross off items from your list to ensure you don't forget anything.

6. **Preparation**: Once you have all the ingredients, set aside some time for meal preparation. Follow the recipes in the cookbook, using the listed ingredients and quantities as your guide.

7. **Cooking**: Cook the recipes according to the provided instructions. Feel free to customize the dishes to suit your taste preferences but try to stay true to the spirit of the recipe.

8. **Enjoy**: Once your meals are cooked, sit down and Savor the fruits of your Labor. Share them with family and friends, and don't forget to appreciate the convenience and variety that your food list cookbook has brought to your table.

9. **Repeat**: Continue exploring new recipes from the cookbook, gradually expanding your culinary skills and experimenting with different Flavors and ingredients

**** The Extra Special Bonuses are after Conclusion****

TABLE OF CONTENTS

INTRODUCTION

Welcome to a journey of culinary delight and health transformation!

I'm Dr. Natalie Pina, a dedicated medical practitioner, and a passionate chef. Join me on an adventure through the world of healing cuisine, where flavour and health intertwine seamlessly.

My journey into the world of healing cuisine started with a simple moment - in my grandmother's kitchen. Surrounded by the comforting aromas of simmering spices and bubbling pots, I discovered the profound connection between food and well-being. These early experiences ignited a flame within me, propelling me toward a career where medicine and gastronomy intersect.

In this comprehensive low cholesterol food list and cookbook, I'll guide you to discover the immense benefits of incorporating low-cholesterol recipes into your lifestyle. But this isn't just any cookbook; it's a guide to transforming your relationship with food. It's about embracing a lifestyle that not only nurtures your body but also tantalizes your taste buds.

As you turn the pages, you'll discover flavourful recipes crafted to promote heart health and overall well-being. This book is not just about food; it's about an experience, a journey toward a healthier, more vibrant you.

Inside, you'll find recipes that nurture your body and evoke a sense of joy and satisfaction. From hearty breakfasts to sumptuous dinners and delightful snacks, this cookbook covers it all. But beyond the recipes, I'll share stories, emotions, and experiences that will resonate with you, inspiring you to take charge of your health and wellness.

Imagine waking up to the aroma of a delicious Spinach and Strawberry Smoothie, knowing that you are starting your day with a burst of flavour and goodness. Picture savouring a Slow Cooker Vegetable Curry, each bite a celebration of health and vitality. Feel the satisfaction of enjoying a Chocolate-Dipped Strawberry, guilt-free, knowing that every ingredient serves your well-being.

But the benefits of this cookbook extend far beyond the delicious recipes. By embracing a low-cholesterol diet, you are taking proactive steps toward a healthier heart and a happier life. You will experience increased energy levels, improved mood, and enhanced overall well-being.

So, whether you are looking to manage your cholesterol levels or simply wish to embark on a journey to better health, this cookbook is your ultimate companion. Join me as we explore the delightful world of healing cuisine together. Let's cook our way to a healthier, happier life, one delicious meal at a time.

Chapter 1
Understanding Cholesterol and Its Impact on Health

Cholesterol is a type of fat found in your blood. While it's often demonized as a health villain, the truth is that cholesterol is essential for your body to function properly. However, having high levels of certain types of cholesterol can increase your risk of heart disease and other health problems.

There are two main types of cholesterol: low-density lipoprotein (LDL) and high-density lipoprotein (HDL). LDL cholesterol is often referred to as "bad" cholesterol because it can build up in the walls of your arteries, leading to atherosclerosis, a condition where your arteries become narrowed and hardened. This can restrict blood flow to vital organs and increase your risk of heart attack and stroke.

On the other hand, HDL cholesterol is often called "good" cholesterol because it helps remove LDL cholesterol from your arteries and carries it back to your liver, where it is broken down and removed from your body. Having higher levels of HDL cholesterol can help protect against heart disease.

Several factors can influence your cholesterol levels, including genetics, diet, exercise, and lifestyle habits. While you can't change your genetics, you can take steps to manage your cholesterol levels and reduce your risk of heart disease. This includes eating a healthy diet that is low in saturated and trans fats, exercising regularly, maintaining a healthy weight, and avoiding smoking.

If you have high cholesterol, your doctor may recommend lifestyle changes and medications to help lower it. Statins are a common type of medication prescribed to lower LDL cholesterol levels. However, it's important to work with your doctor to find the right treatment plan for you, as medications can have side effects and may not be suitable for everyone.

Regular cholesterol screenings are also important for monitoring your cholesterol levels and assessing your risk of heart disease. Your doctor can recommend how often you should be tested based on your age, family history, and other risk factors.

Benefits of a Low Cholesterol Diet

Following a low cholesterol diet can offer numerous health benefits, especially in reducing the risk of heart disease and promoting overall well-being. Here are some of the key advantages:

1. Heart Health: One of the primary benefits of a low cholesterol diet is its positive impact on heart health. By reducing the intake of cholesterol-rich foods, such as fatty meats, full-fat dairy products, and processed snacks, you can lower levels of LDL cholesterol, the type of cholesterol associated with an increased risk of heart disease. This, in turn, helps to prevent the buildup of plaque in the arteries and reduces the risk of heart attacks and strokes.

2. Improved Blood Circulation: A diet low in cholesterol also supports better blood circulation throughout the body. When LDL cholesterol levels are high, it can lead to atherosclerosis, a condition characterized by the narrowing and hardening of arteries due to the buildup of plaque. By adopting a low cholesterol diet, you can help keep your arteries clear and promote healthy blood flow, which is essential for delivering oxygen and nutrients to all parts of the body.

3. Weight Management: Many foods high in cholesterol are also high in saturated fats and calories, which can contribute to weight gain and obesity.

By choosing low cholesterol alternatives, such as fruits, vegetables, whole grains, and lean proteins, you can reduce your calorie intake and support weight management efforts. Maintaining a healthy weight is important for reducing the risk of numerous health conditions, including heart disease, diabetes, and certain types of cancer.

4. Lower Blood Pressure: High cholesterol levels can contribute to high blood pressure, another major risk factor for heart disease. By following a low cholesterol diet that emphasizes whole, nutrient-rich foods and limits processed and high-sodium options, you can help keep your blood pressure within a healthy range. This can further reduce the strain on your heart and lower the risk of cardiovascular problems.

5. Better Overall Health: Beyond its impact on heart health, a low cholesterol diet can promote overall well-being. By focusing on whole foods that are rich in vitamins, minerals, and antioxidants, you provide your body with the nutrients it needs to function optimally. Additionally, such a diet can help reduce inflammation in the body, strengthen the immune system, and support digestive health.

Tips for Lowering Cholesterol Through Diet

Lowering cholesterol through diet is an effective way to improve heart health and reduce the risk of cardiovascular disease. Here are some practical tips to help you lower your cholesterol levels:

1. Choose Heart-Healthy Fats: Replace saturated and trans fats with healthier fats, such as monounsaturated and polyunsaturated fats. Opt for sources like olive oil, avocado, nuts, seeds, and fatty fish like salmon and mackerel. These fats can help raise HDL (good) cholesterol levels and lower LDL (bad) cholesterol levels.

2. Increase Fiber Intake: Include plenty of soluble fiber in your diet, as it can help lower LDL cholesterol levels. Good sources of soluble fiber include oats, barley, beans, lentils, fruits, and vegetables. Aim for at least 25-30 grams of fiber per day.

3. Eat More Plant-Based Foods: Plant-based foods like fruits, vegetables, whole grains, legumes, and nuts are naturally low in cholesterol and saturated fats. They're also rich in fiber, antioxidants, and other nutrients that support heart health. Try to make plant-based meals the focus of your diet.

4. Limit Animal Products: Reduce your intake of high-cholesterol animal products, such as fatty meats, processed meats, and full-fat dairy products. Choose lean cuts of meat, skinless poultry, and low-fat dairy alternatives instead. Limit your consumption of red meat and opt for leaner protein sources more often.

5. Watch Portion Sizes: Be mindful of portion sizes, especially when it comes to high-calorie and high-fat foods. Even healthy fats can contribute to

weight gain if consumed in excess. Use smaller plates, measure serving sizes, and avoid oversized portions to help control your calorie intake.

6. Choose Low-Fat Cooking Methods: Opt for cooking methods that require little or no added fat, such as grilling, baking, steaming, and broiling. Use herbs, spices, and citrus juices to add flavor to your dishes instead of relying on butter or oil.

7. Be Selective with Snacks: Choose heart-healthy snacks like fresh fruits, vegetables with hummus, air-popped popcorn, or a handful of nuts. Avoid processed snacks that are high in saturated fats, trans fats, and cholesterol.

8. Be Mindful of Hidden Fats: Pay attention to hidden sources of fats and cholesterol in packaged and processed foods, such as fried foods, pastries, commercial baked goods, and snack foods. Read food labels carefully and choose products with lower amounts of saturated and trans fats.

9. Stay Hydrated: Drink plenty of water throughout the day to stay hydrated and support overall health. Limit sugary beverages, alcohol, and drinks high in saturated fats, such as creamy coffee drinks.

10. Be Consistent: Remember that making dietary changes takes time and consistency. Focus on making small, sustainable changes to your eating habits and stick with them over the long term for lasting results.

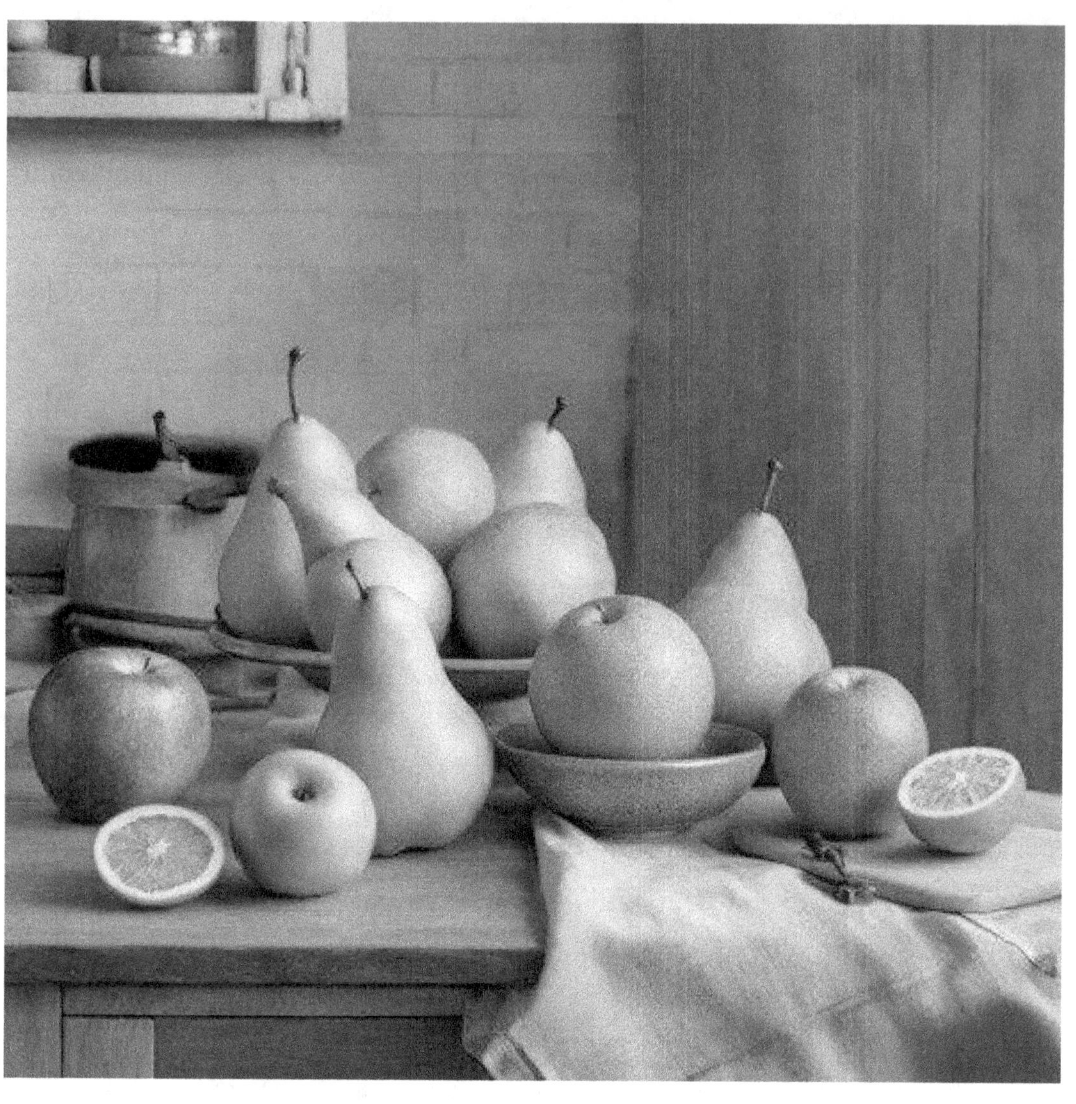

Chapter 2:
Building a Low-Cholesterol Pantry

Creating a low-cholesterol pantry is an essential step toward managing cholesterol levels and promoting heart health. By filling your pantry with wholesome, cholesterol-friendly foods, you can make it easier to prepare delicious and heart-conscious meals at home. Here are some tips for building a low-cholesterol pantry:

1. **Whole Grains**: Stock up on whole grains such as brown rice, quinoa, barley, oats, whole wheat pasta, and whole grain bread. These foods are high in fiber and nutrients, which can help lower LDL (bad) cholesterol levels and reduce the risk of heart disease.

2. **Legumes**: Include a variety of legumes in your pantry, such as lentils, beans, chickpeas, and peas. Legumes are excellent sources of plant-based protein, fiber, and nutrients, and they can help lower cholesterol and improve heart health.

3. **Nuts and Seeds**: Keep unsalted nuts and seeds like almonds, walnuts, flaxseeds, chia seeds, and pumpkin seeds on hand. These foods are rich in heart-healthy fats, fiber, and antioxidants, and they can help lower LDL cholesterol levels.

4. **Healthy Oils**: Choose heart-healthy oils such as olive oil, avocado oil, and canola oil for cooking and salad dressings. These oils are low in saturated fats and high in monounsaturated and polyunsaturated fats, which can help improve cholesterol levels and support heart health.

5. **Lean Proteins**: Opt for lean protein sources such as skinless poultry, fish, tofu, tempeh, and legumes. Limit your intake of high-cholesterol animal products like fatty meats and full-fat dairy products.

6. **Low-Fat Dairy Alternatives**: Choose low-fat or fat-free dairy alternatives such as skim milk, unsweetened almond milk, and low-fat yogurt. These options are lower in saturated fats and cholesterol compared to full-fat dairy products.

7. **Herbs and Spices**: Use herbs, spices, and seasonings to add flavor to your meals without adding extra salt or unhealthy fats. Keep a variety of herbs and spices on hand, such as garlic, turmeric, cinnamon, basil, oregano, and thyme.

8. **Fresh Fruits and Vegetables**: Stock your pantry with a variety of fresh fruits and vegetables, as well as frozen and canned options without added sugars or sauces. These foods are rich in fiber, vitamins, minerals, and antioxidants, which can help lower cholesterol and support heart health.

9. **Whole Grain Snacks**: Keep heart-healthy snacks on hand for when hunger strikes between meals. Choose whole grain crackers, air-popped popcorn, rice cakes, and whole grain cereal bars for satisfying and nutritious options.

10. **Low-Cholesterol Cooking Ingredients**: Choose low-cholesterol cooking ingredients such as egg substitutes, cholesterol-free margarine, and cholesterol-lowering spreads. These options can help reduce cholesterol intake while still enjoying your favorite recipes.

Smart Shopping Tips for Low-Cholesterol Foods

Making smart choices at the grocery store is essential for maintaining a low-cholesterol diet and supporting heart health. Here are some tips to help you shop for low-cholesterol foods:

1. **Plan**: Before heading to the store, make a list of low-cholesterol foods and meals you want to prepare for the week. Planning can help you stay focused and avoid impulse purchases of high-cholesterol items.

2. **Read Food Labels**: Take the time to read food labels carefully and look for products that are low in cholesterol and saturated fats. Pay attention to serving sizes and the cholesterol content per serving. Choose options with lower cholesterol and saturated fat levels whenever possible.

3. **Focus on Whole Foods**: Shop the perimeter of the grocery store where fresh produce, lean proteins, and whole grains are typically located. Choose whole foods like fruits, vegetables, whole grains, and lean meats to build a nutritious and low-cholesterol diet.

4. **Choose Lean Proteins**: When selecting meats, opt for lean cuts like skinless poultry, fish, and lean cuts of beef or pork. Trim visible fat from meat and remove the skin from poultry to reduce cholesterol and saturated fat intake.

5. **Include Plant-Based Proteins**: Incorporate plant-based protein sources like beans, lentils, chickpeas, and tofu into your meals. These options are low in cholesterol and saturated fat and rich in fiber and nutrients that support heart health.

6. **Select Low-Fat Dairy**: Choose low-fat or fat-free dairy products such as skim milk, yogurt, and cheese to reduce cholesterol and saturated fat intake.

Look for options labeled "low-fat" or "fat-free" and avoid products with added sugars or flavors.

7. **Opt for Whole Grains**: Stock up on whole grain options like brown rice, quinoa, oats, and whole wheat pasta and bread. These foods are high in fiber and nutrients and can help lower LDL (bad) cholesterol levels.

8. **Limit Processed Foods**: Minimize your intake of processed and packaged foods that are often high in cholesterol, saturated fats, and added sugars. Instead, focus on whole, minimally processed foods that are naturally low in cholesterol and rich in nutrients.

9. **Choose Healthy Fats**: Incorporate heart-healthy fats like olive oil, avocado, nuts, and seeds into your diet in moderation. These fats can help raise HDL (good) cholesterol levels and improve overall heart health.

10. **Shop Seasonally and Locally**: Take advantage of seasonal produce and local farmers' markets to find fresh, affordable, and nutritious options. Seasonal fruits and vegetables are often at their peak flavor and nutritional value.

Reading Food Labels for Cholesterol Content

Understanding how to read food labels is essential for managing your cholesterol intake and making informed choices about the foods you eat. Here's a guide to help you interpret food labels for cholesterol content:

1. **Check the Serving Size**: Start by looking at the serving size listed on the food label. All the information on the label, including cholesterol content, is based on this serving size. Be mindful of portion sizes to accurately assess your cholesterol intake.

2. **Identify Total Cholesterol**: Look for the total cholesterol content listed on the label. This value represents the amount of cholesterol in one serving of the food product. Aim to choose foods with lower total cholesterol levels.

3. **Review % Daily Value (%DV)**: The %DV indicates how much of a particular nutrient, such as cholesterol, one serving of the food contributes to your daily recommended intake. As a general guideline, aim for foods with a %DV of 5% or less for cholesterol. Foods with 20% or more of the %DV for cholesterol are considered high in cholesterol.

4. **Check for Saturated Fat and Trans Fat**: While not directly related to cholesterol intake, saturated and trans fats can raise LDL (bad) cholesterol levels. Choose foods that are low in saturated and trans fats to help manage cholesterol levels. Keep in mind that some labels may list cholesterol-free products that still contain unhealthy fats.

5. **Look for Health Claims**: Some food labels may include health claims related to cholesterol, such as "low cholesterol" or "cholesterol-free." While these claims can be helpful, it's essential to review the nutrition facts panel

to verify the cholesterol content and assess other nutritional aspects of the food.

6. **Compare Similar Products**: When shopping for packaged foods, compare similar products to find the option with the lowest cholesterol content. Pay attention to differences in serving sizes and %DV to make accurate comparisons.

7. **Consider Other Nutrients**: In addition to cholesterol, consider other nutrients listed on the food label, such as fiber, vitamins, and minerals. Choosing foods that are high in fiber and nutrients can support heart health and overall well-being.

8. **Be Mindful of Hidden Sources**: Keep in mind that cholesterol can be found in unexpected sources, such as processed foods, baked goods, and dairy products. Read ingredient lists carefully to identify hidden sources of cholesterol and make informed choices.

9. **Focus on Whole Foods**: Whenever possible, choose whole, minimally processed foods that are naturally low in cholesterol. Fruits, vegetables, whole grains, lean proteins, and plant-based foods are excellent choices for managing cholesterol intake and supporting heart health.

10. **Consult with a Healthcare Professional**: If you have specific dietary restrictions or health concerns related to cholesterol, consider consulting with a healthcare professional or registered dietitian for personalized guidance and recommendations.

Chapter 3
Low Cholesterol Fruits &
Fruits to Avoid

1. **Berries (Strawberries, Blueberries, Raspberries, Blackberries):**

   - Nutritional Information: Berries are low in calories and high in fiber, antioxidants, and various vitamins like vitamin C and K. For instance, a cup of strawberries contains about 50 calories and provides over 100% of the recommended daily intake of vitamin C.

   - Explanation: Berries are excellent low-cholesterol fruit options due to their high fiber content, which helps in lowering cholesterol levels and improving heart health. Additionally, their antioxidants help fight inflammation and oxidative stress.

2. **Apples:**

   - Nutritional Information: Apples are rich in dietary fiber, particularly pectin, along with vitamin C and various antioxidants. A medium-sized apple contains around 95 calories and provides about 4 grams of fiber.

   - Explanation: The soluble fiber found in apples, especially in their skin, helps lower LDL cholesterol levels (the "bad" cholesterol) by reducing its absorption in the bloodstream. Regular consumption of apples can contribute to better heart health.

3. **Pears:**

- Nutritional Information: Pears are another excellent source of dietary fiber, vitamins C and K, as well as antioxidants like flavonoids. A medium-sized pear contains approximately 100 calories and provides about 5 grams of fiber.

- Explanation: Like apples, pears contain soluble fiber, particularly in their skin, which aids in lowering cholesterol levels. Including pears in your diet can support digestive health and contribute to overall well-being.

4. **Oranges:**

- Nutritional Information: Oranges are famous for their high vitamin C content and also provide dietary fiber, potassium, and various antioxidants. A medium-sized orange contains around 60 calories and offers about 3 grams of fiber.

- Explanation: Oranges are low in calories and cholesterol-free, making them a heart-healthy choice. The soluble fiber in oranges, primarily found in their pulp, helps reduce cholesterol levels by binding with bile acids in the gut and promoting their excretion.

5. **Kiwi:**

- Nutritional Information: Kiwifruit is rich in vitamin C, vitamin K, dietary fiber, and antioxidants like vitamin E and polyphenols. A medium-sized kiwi contains approximately 50 calories and provides around 2.5 grams of fiber.

- Explanation: Kiwis are not only delicious but also contribute to heart health due to their high fiber content. The soluble fiber in kiwifruit can help lower LDL cholesterol levels, while its antioxidants combat inflammation and oxidative stress, further supporting cardiovascular health.

6. **Grapes:**

- Nutritional Information: Grapes are rich in antioxidants, particularly resveratrol, along with vitamin C and potassium. A cup of grapes contains around 60-70 calories and provides about 1 gram of fiber.

- Explanation: Grapes help support heart health by improving circulation and reducing inflammation. The antioxidants in grapes, especially in red and purple varieties, can help lower LDL cholesterol levels and protect against cardiovascular diseases.

7. **Bananas:**

- Nutritional Information: Bananas are a good source of potassium, vitamin B6, vitamin C, and dietary fiber. A medium-sized banana contains approximately 100-110 calories and provides about 3 grams of fiber.

- Explanation: Despite their slightly higher calorie content compared to some other fruits, bananas are still considered low in cholesterol and beneficial for heart health. The soluble fiber in bananas helps lower cholesterol levels and regulate blood sugar levels, making them a nutritious choice for snacks and breakfast.

8. **Peaches:**

- Nutritional Information: Peaches are rich in vitamins A and C, as well as dietary fiber and antioxidants like beta-carotene and lutein. A medium-sized peach contains about 60-70 calories and provides around 2 grams of fiber.

- Explanation: Peaches are not only delicious but also contribute to lowering cholesterol levels and supporting heart health. The fiber and antioxidants in peaches help reduce LDL cholesterol oxidation and inflammation, which are crucial factors in preventing cardiovascular diseases.

9. **Plums:**

- Nutritional Information: Plums are high in vitamins C and K, dietary fiber, and antioxidants like phenolic compounds. A medium-sized plum contains approximately 30-40 calories and provides about 1 gram of fiber.

- Explanation: Plums are low in cholesterol and provide various health benefits, including supporting heart health. The soluble fiber in plums helps lower LDL cholesterol levels, while their antioxidants protect against oxidative stress and inflammation, reducing the risk of heart diseases.

10. **Cherries:**

- Nutritional Information: Cherries are packed with antioxidants, particularly anthocyanins, as well as vitamins C and K, and dietary fiber. A cup of cherries contains around 80-90 calories and provides about 3 grams of fiber.

- Explanation: Cherries are not only low in cholesterol but also help improve heart health due to their anti-inflammatory and antioxidant properties. Regular consumption of cherries can help lower LDL cholesterol levels, reduce inflammation, and decrease the risk of cardiovascular diseases.

Fruits to Avoid

1. **Avocado:**

    *   While fruits typically don't contain cholesterol, avocados are unique in that they are high in healthy fats, particularly monounsaturated fats. While these fats are beneficial for heart health in moderation, they can contribute to higher cholesterol levels if consumed excessively. However, it's important to note that the fats in avocados are mostly healthy fats that can actually help raise HDL (good) cholesterol levels while lowering LDL (bad) cholesterol.

2. **Coconut:**

    *   Coconut, including its meat and oil, contains saturated fats, which can raise LDL cholesterol levels when consumed in large amounts. Coconut products are versatile and commonly used in cooking and baking, but moderation is key due to their potential impact on cholesterol levels.

3. **Durian:**

    *   Durian is a tropical fruit known for its distinctive odor and creamy texture. It contains both saturated and unsaturated fats, which can contribute to higher cholesterol levels if consumed excessively. Like other high-fat fruits, enjoying durian in moderation is advisable for individuals concerned about their cholesterol levels.

4. **Palm Fruit:**

    *   Palm fruit and its oil are commonly used in cooking and food processing. Palm oil, in particular, contains a high amount of saturated fats, which can raise LDL cholesterol levels when

consumed in excess. While palm fruit itself may not be widely consumed in its fresh form, its oil is prevalent in many processed foods.

5. **Cacao (Chocolate):**

   - Cacao beans, from which chocolate is made, contain cocoa butter, which is high in saturated fats. While dark chocolate does offer some health benefits due to its antioxidants, consuming it excessively can contribute to higher cholesterol levels due to its saturated fat content.

Explanation: These fruits, while naturally cholesterol-free, can contribute to higher cholesterol levels due to their high content of saturated or unhealthy fats. Saturated fats can raise LDL (bad) cholesterol levels, increasing the risk of heart disease if consumed in excess. However, it's essential to remember that moderation is key, and these fruits can still be part of a healthy diet when consumed in appropriate portions as part of a balanced diet.

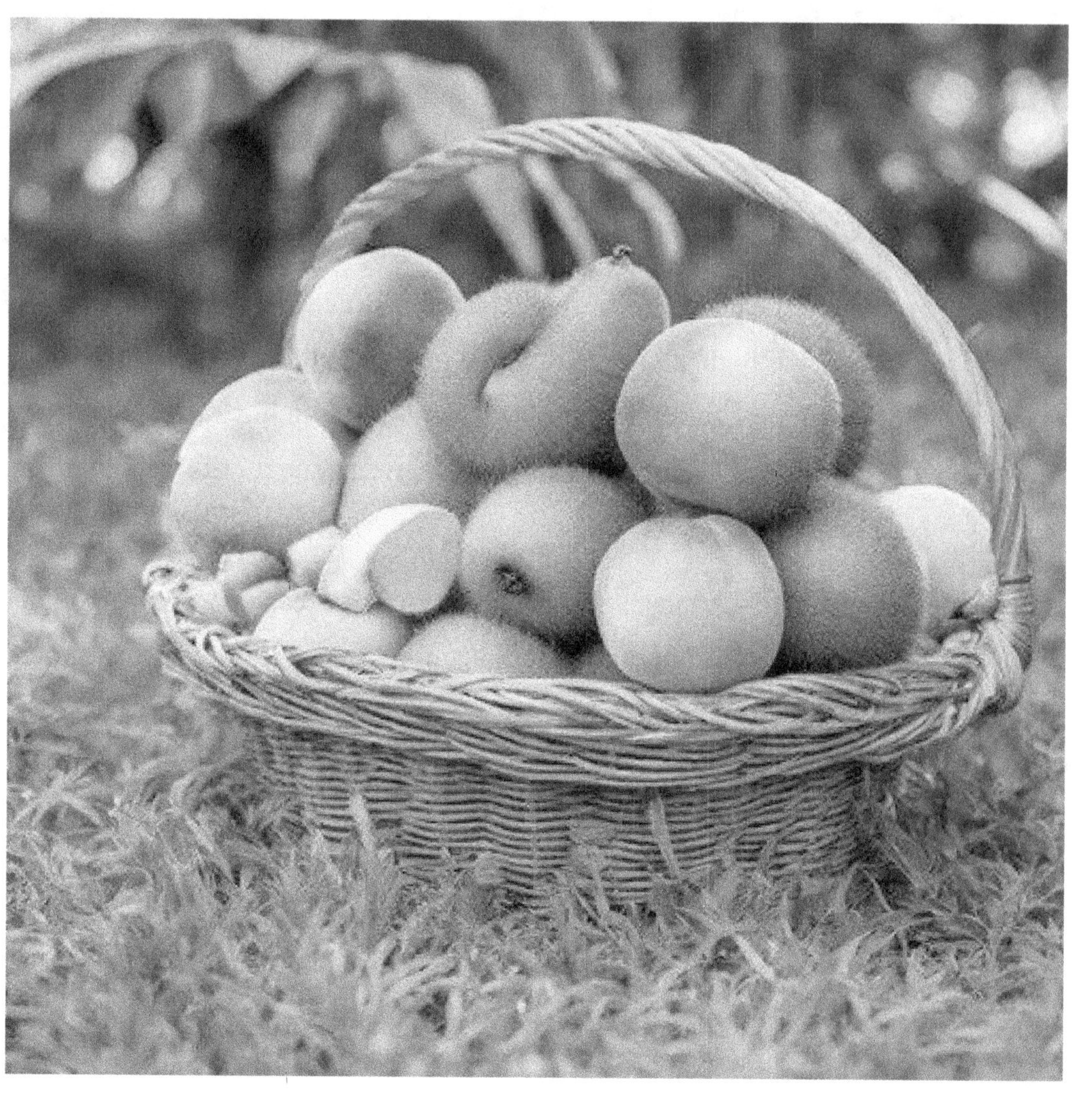

Chapter 4: Low Cholesterol Vegetables & Veggies to Avoid

1. **Spinach:**

   - Nutritional Information: Spinach is rich in vitamins A, C, and K, as well as folate, iron, and calcium. One cup of raw spinach contains only about 7 calories and provides nearly 200% of the daily recommended intake of vitamin K.

   - Explanation: Spinach is a nutrient-dense leafy green vegetable that is low in calories and cholesterol-free. It is high in fiber, which helps lower cholesterol levels and promotes digestive health.

2. **Broccoli:**

   - Nutritional Information: Broccoli is packed with vitamins C and K, as well as folate, fiber, and antioxidants like sulforaphane. One cup of chopped broccoli contains about 30 calories and provides over 100% of the daily recommended intake of vitamin C.

   - Explanation: Broccoli is a cruciferous vegetable known for its cholesterol-lowering properties. It contains soluble fiber, which binds to cholesterol in the digestive tract, preventing its absorption into the bloodstream.

3. **Bell Peppers:**

   - Nutritional Information: Bell peppers are rich in vitamins A, C, and K, as well as potassium and antioxidants like beta-carotene. One medium-sized bell pepper contains about 30 calories and provides over 100% of the daily recommended intake of vitamin C.

- Explanation: Bell peppers are low in calories and cholesterol-free, making them a heart-healthy vegetable choice. Their high vitamin C content helps lower LDL cholesterol levels and reduce the risk of cardiovascular diseases.

4. **Cauliflower:**

- Nutritional Information: Cauliflower is high in vitamins C and K, as well as folate, fiber, and antioxidants like glucosinolates. One cup of chopped cauliflower contains about 25 calories and provides over 75% of the daily recommended intake of vitamin C.

- Explanation: Cauliflower is a versatile vegetable that can be used as a low-carb substitute for grains and legumes. It contains soluble fiber, which helps lower cholesterol levels and promotes satiety, making it beneficial for weight management.

5. **Carrots:**

- Nutritional Information: Carrots are rich in beta-carotene, vitamins A, K, and B6, as well as fiber and potassium. One medium-sized carrot contains about 25 calories and provides over 200% of the daily recommended intake of vitamin A.

- Explanation: Carrots are low in calories and cholesterol-free, making them a healthy addition to any diet. Their high fiber content helps lower cholesterol levels and improve digestive health.

6. **Zucchini:**

- Nutritional Information: Zucchini is low in calories and high in water content, making it hydrating and nutrient-rich. One cup of sliced zucchini contains about 20 calories and provides over 10% of the daily recommended intake of vitamin C.

- Explanation: Zucchini is a versatile vegetable that can be enjoyed raw or cooked in various dishes. It is low in cholesterol and high in fiber, which helps lower cholesterol levels and promote feelings of fullness.

7. **Kale:**

- Nutritional Information: Kale is a nutrient-dense leafy green vegetable high in vitamins A, C, and K, as well as calcium, iron, and antioxidants like lutein and zeaxanthin. One cup of chopped kale contains about 35 calories and provides over 100% of the daily recommended intake of vitamin A.

- Explanation: Kale is known for its cholesterol-lowering properties due to its high fiber content. It also contains antioxidants that help reduce inflammation and oxidative stress, promoting overall heart health.

8. **Cabbage:**

- Nutritional Information: Cabbage is low in calories and high in fiber, vitamins C and K, and antioxidants like sulforaphane. One cup of shredded cabbage contains about 20 calories and provides over 50% of the daily recommended intake of vitamin C.

- Explanation: Cabbage is a cruciferous vegetable with cholesterol-lowering properties. Its high fiber content helps reduce LDL cholesterol levels and improve digestive health, making it beneficial for overall well-being.

9. **Asparagus:**

- Nutritional Information: Asparagus is rich in vitamins A, C, and K, as well as folate, fiber, and antioxidants like glutathione. One cup of cooked asparagus contains about 40 calories and provides over 60% of the daily recommended intake of vitamin K.

- Explanation: Asparagus is a low-calorie vegetable with cholesterol-lowering properties. It contains soluble fiber, which helps reduce LDL cholesterol levels and promotes cardiovascular health.

10. **Cucumber:**

- Nutritional Information: Cucumber is high in water content and low in calories, making it refreshing and hydrating. One cup of sliced cucumber contains about 15 calories and provides over 10% of the daily recommended intake of vitamin K.

- Explanation: Cucumber is a cholesterol-free vegetable that is often enjoyed raw in salads and sandwiches. Its high water and fiber content promote hydration and digestive health, making it an excellent choice for weight management and overall well-being.

Veggies to Avoid

1. **Coconut**:

   - While technically a fruit, coconut is often used in savory dishes and contains saturated fats. Consuming coconut in various forms, such as coconut meat or coconut oil, can contribute to higher cholesterol levels due to its saturated fat content.

2. **Palm Hearts**:

   - Palm hearts, harvested from the inner core of certain palm trees, are relatively low in calories but contain a small amount of saturated fat. While not a significant source of cholesterol themselves, dishes containing palm hearts may contribute to higher cholesterol intake if prepared with added fats or oils.

3. **Canned Vegetables in Oil**:

   - Certain canned vegetables, particularly those preserved in oil, may contain added saturated fats, contributing to higher cholesterol intake. Vegetables like artichokes, sun-dried tomatoes, or peppers preserved in oil should be consumed in moderation to avoid excess saturated fat intake.

4. **Cassava/Yuca**:

   - Cassava, a starchy root vegetable popular in many cuisines, contains minimal fat but is high in carbohydrates. While not directly contributing to cholesterol levels, consuming cassava-based dishes that are fried or prepared with added fats can indirectly impact cholesterol levels due to the added saturated fats from cooking oils.

5. **Plantain**:

- Plantains, a starchy fruit commonly used in savory dishes, are naturally low in fat but can absorb significant amounts of oil when fried or cooked in oil-based sauces. Consuming plantains in dishes prepared with excessive amounts of oil can contribute to higher cholesterol intake due to the added saturated fats.

Explanation: While vegetables are typically low in cholesterol, certain preparation methods or accompanying ingredients can lead to higher cholesterol intake. Foods prepared with saturated fats, such as coconut oil or palm oil, can raise LDL (bad) cholesterol levels when consumed in excess. Therefore, it's essential to be mindful of cooking methods and ingredients to maintain a heart-healthy diet. Opting for cooking techniques like baking, grilling, steaming, or sautéing with healthier fats like olive oil can help reduce the intake of saturated fats and promote better cholesterol levels.

Chapter 5
Low Cholesterol lean Protein & Protein to Avoid

1. **Chicken Breast:**

    - Nutritional Information: A 3-ounce serving of cooked chicken breast provides about 165 calories, 31 grams of protein, and minimal fat.

    - Explanation: Chicken breast is a lean protein source that is low in cholesterol and saturated fat. It's versatile, easy to cook, and can be incorporated into various dishes while providing essential amino acids for muscle building and repair.

2. **Turkey Breast:**

    - Nutritional Information: A 3-ounce serving of cooked turkey breast contains approximately 125 calories, 26 grams of protein, and minimal fat.

    - Explanation: Similar to chicken breast, turkey breast is a lean protein option that is low in cholesterol and saturated fat. It's a nutritious choice for those looking to maintain or improve their cholesterol levels while meeting their protein needs.

3. **Fish (Cod):**

    - Nutritional Information: A 3-ounce serving of cooked cod provides about 90 calories, 20 grams of protein, and less than 1 gram of fat.

- Explanation: Cod is a lean white fish that is low in cholesterol and saturated fat. It's an excellent source of high-quality protein and omega-3 fatty acids, which have been shown to support heart health and lower cholesterol levels.

4. **Tofu:**

- Nutritional Information: A 3-ounce serving of firm tofu contains approximately 70 calories, 8 grams of protein, and 4 grams of fat.

- Explanation: Tofu is a plant-based protein option made from soybeans and is naturally cholesterol-free. It's rich in protein, low in saturated fat, and can be used in a variety of dishes as a meat alternative for those following a vegetarian or vegan diet.

5. **Egg Whites:**

- Nutritional Information: Two large egg whites provide about 34 calories, 7 grams of protein, and less than 1 gram of fat.

- Explanation: Egg whites are a low-cholesterol, high-protein option that can be used in cooking and baking. They are cholesterol-free and contain essential amino acids necessary for muscle maintenance and repair.

6. **Lentils:**

- Nutritional Information: A 1/2 cup serving of cooked lentils contains approximately 115 calories, 9 grams of protein, and less than 1 gram of fat.

- Explanation: Lentils are a plant-based protein source that is low in cholesterol and saturated fat. They are also high in fiber, vitamins, and minerals, making them a heart-healthy choice for those looking to lower their cholesterol levels.

7. **Skinless Turkey or Chicken Sausage:**

   - Nutritional Information: A 2-ounce serving of skinless turkey or chicken sausage provides about 100-150 calories, 10-15 grams of protein, and varying amounts of fat depending on the brand.

   - Explanation: Opting for skinless turkey or chicken sausage can be a lower-fat alternative to traditional pork sausage. They are lower in cholesterol and saturated fat while still providing a good amount of protein.

8. **Greek Yogurt:**

   - Nutritional Information: A 6-ounce serving of plain Greek yogurt contains approximately 100 calories, 17 grams of protein, and 0-3 grams of fat depending on the fat content.

   - Explanation: Greek yogurt is a high-protein dairy option that is lower in cholesterol and saturated fat compared to other dairy products like cheese or cream. It's rich in probiotics, calcium, and other nutrients beneficial for gut and bone health.

9. **Beans (Black Beans, Chickpeas, Kidney Beans):**

   - Nutritional Information: A 1/2 cup serving of cooked beans provides about 110-120 calories, 7-8 grams of protein, and less than 1 gram of fat.

   - Explanation: Beans are a cholesterol-free source of plant-based protein that is also high in fiber, vitamins, and minerals. They can be incorporated into soups, salads, and main dishes for a nutritious boost.

10. **Soy Milk:**

- Nutritional Information: A 1-cup serving of unsweetened soy milk contains approximately 80-90 calories, 7-9 grams of protein, and 4-4.5 grams of fat.

- Explanation: Soy milk is a dairy-free alternative to cow's milk that is naturally cholesterol-free and low in saturated fat. It's fortified with calcium, vitamin D, and other nutrients, making it a suitable option for those with lactose intolerance or following a vegan diet.

Incorporating these low-cholesterol lean protein sources into your diet can help support heart health and maintain healthy cholesterol levels while providing essential nutrients for overall well-being.

Protein to Avoid

1. **Organ Meats (Liver, Kidneys, Heart):**

   - Organ meats are rich in cholesterol, with liver being one of the highest cholesterol-containing foods. They also tend to be higher in saturated fats compared to lean cuts of meat. Consuming organ meats can contribute to higher cholesterol levels, particularly LDL (bad) cholesterol.

2. **Shellfish (Shrimp, Lobster, Crab):**

   - While shellfish are low in saturated fat, they are relatively high in cholesterol. For example, a 3-ounce serving of shrimp contains about 166 milligrams of cholesterol. While they can be part of a healthy diet, individuals with high cholesterol levels may need to moderate their intake of shellfish.

3. **Processed Meats (Bacon, Sausage, Hot Dogs):**

   - Processed meats are often high in both cholesterol and saturated fats. Additionally, they may contain additives like nitrates and preservatives, which have been linked to increased risk of heart disease. Consuming processed meats regularly can contribute to higher cholesterol levels and other cardiovascular risk factors.

4. **Fatty Cuts of Meat (Ribeye Steak, T-Bone Steak):**

   - Fatty cuts of meat are higher in both cholesterol and saturated fats compared to lean cuts. For example, a 3-ounce serving of ribeye steak contains about 70 milligrams of cholesterol and 4.5 grams of saturated fat. Regular consumption of fatty cuts of meat can raise LDL (bad) cholesterol levels and increase the risk of heart disease.

5. **Full-Fat Dairy Products (Whole Milk, Cheese, Butter):**

- Full-fat dairy products contain cholesterol and saturated fats, which can contribute to higher cholesterol levels when consumed in excess. For example, a 1-ounce serving of cheddar cheese contains about 29 milligrams of cholesterol and 6 grams of saturated fat. Choosing low-fat or fat-free dairy options can help lower cholesterol intake.

Explanation: These protein sources tend to be higher in cholesterol and/or saturated fats, both of which can raise LDL (bad) cholesterol levels and increase the risk of heart disease when consumed in excess. While they can still be part of a balanced diet in moderation, it's important for individuals with high cholesterol levels or cardiovascular risk factors to be mindful of their intake of these protein sources and opt for leaner, lower-cholesterol alternatives more often.

Chapter 6: Low Cholesterol Whole Grain and Fiber

& Grain and Fiber to Avoid

1. **Oats:**

   - Nutritional Information: A 1/2 cup serving of cooked oats contains approximately 150 calories, 3 grams of fat, 27 grams of carbohydrates, 4 grams of fiber, and 5 grams of protein.

   - Explanation: Oats are a whole grain rich in soluble fiber, which helps lower LDL (bad) cholesterol levels. They are also a good source of complex carbohydrates, providing sustained energy and promoting digestive health.

2. **Quinoa:**

   - Nutritional Information: A 1/2 cup serving of cooked quinoa provides around 111 calories, 2 grams of fat, 20 grams of carbohydrates, 2.6 grams of fiber, and 4 grams of protein.

   - Explanation: Quinoa is a complete protein source and a gluten-free whole grain that is high in fiber. Its fiber content aids in digestion and helps regulate cholesterol levels, making it a heart-healthy choice.

3. **Brown Rice:**

- Nutritional Information: A 1/2 cup serving of cooked brown rice contains approximately 108 calories, 1 gram of fat, 22 grams of carbohydrates, 1.8 grams of fiber, and 2.3 grams of protein.

- Explanation: Brown rice is a whole grain that retains its bran and germ layers, making it rich in fiber and nutrients. Its fiber content promotes satiety, aids in digestion, and helps lower cholesterol levels.

4. **Barley:**

- Nutritional Information: A 1/2 cup serving of cooked barley provides about 97 calories, 0.5 grams of fat, 22 grams of carbohydrates, 3.5 grams of fiber, and 2.5 grams of protein.

- Explanation: Barley is high in soluble fiber, particularly beta-glucan, which has been shown to reduce LDL cholesterol levels. It also contains antioxidants and other nutrients that support heart health.

5. **Whole Wheat Pasta:**

- Nutritional Information: A 1/2 cup serving of cooked whole wheat pasta contains approximately 97 calories, 0.8 grams of fat, 20 grams of carbohydrates, 3.5 grams of fiber, and 4 grams of protein.

- Explanation: Whole wheat pasta is made from whole grain durum wheat flour, retaining its fiber and nutrient content. Its fiber aids in digestion and helps regulate cholesterol levels, making it a healthier alternative to refined pasta.

6. **Bulgur:**

- Nutritional Information: A 1/2 cup serving of cooked bulgur provides about 76 calories, 0.2 grams of fat, 17 grams of carbohydrates, 4.2 grams of fiber, and 3 grams of protein.

- Explanation: Bulgur is a quick-cooking whole grain made from cracked wheat. It is high in fiber, which promotes digestive health and helps lower cholesterol levels, making it a nutritious addition to salads, soups, and pilafs.

7. **Millet:**

- Nutritional Information: A 1/2 cup serving of cooked millet contains approximately 104 calories, 1.7 grams of fat, 20 grams of carbohydrates, 1.7 grams of fiber, and 3.9 grams of protein.

- Explanation: Millet is a gluten-free whole grain that is high in fiber and rich in nutrients like magnesium and phosphorus. Its fiber content aids in digestion and helps maintain healthy cholesterol levels.

8. **Whole Grain Bread (100% Whole Wheat):**

- Nutritional Information: One slice of 100% whole wheat bread provides around 70-80 calories, 1 gram of fat, 12-14 grams of carbohydrates, 2-3 grams of fiber, and 3-4 grams of protein.

- Explanation: Whole wheat bread is made from whole grain wheat flour, providing fiber and nutrients that promote digestive health and help regulate cholesterol levels. Choosing whole grain bread over refined white bread can contribute to a healthier diet.

9. **Farro:**

- Nutritional Information: A 1/2 cup serving of cooked farro contains approximately 100 calories, 0.5 grams of fat, 20 grams of carbohydrates, 3 grams of fiber, and 4 grams of protein.

- Explanation: Farro is an ancient whole grain that is high in fiber, protein, and nutrients like magnesium and iron. Its fiber content aids in digestion and helps lower cholesterol levels, making it a nutritious addition to salads, soups, and grain bowls.

10. **Buckwheat:**

- Nutritional Information: A 1/2 cup serving of cooked buckwheat provides about 75 calories, 0.5 grams of fat, 17 grams of carbohydrates, 1.5 grams of fiber, and 3 grams of protein.

- Explanation: Buckwheat is a gluten-free whole grain that is rich in fiber and antioxidants like rutin. Its fiber content supports digestive health and helps regulate cholesterol levels, making it a healthy choice for grain-based dishes.

Incorporating these low-cholesterol whole grain and fiber-rich foods into your diet can help improve heart health, regulate cholesterol levels, and promote overall well-being.

Whole and Fiber to Avoid

High-cholesterol whole grain and fiber-rich foods are not common, as whole grains and fiber are typically associated with heart-healthy diets that aim to lower cholesterol levels. However, some processed or refined grain products may contain added fats or sugars that could contribute to higher cholesterol levels. Here are a few examples:

1. **Certain Commercial Granola Bars:**

   - Explanation: While some granola bars are made with whole grains and fiber-rich ingredients like oats and nuts, others may contain added sugars, hydrogenated oils, or high-fructose corn syrup to enhance flavor or texture. These additives can contribute to higher cholesterol levels, particularly if consumed frequently as part of a diet high in saturated fats and sugars.

2. **Packaged Baked Goods (Muffins, Pastries):**

   - Explanation: Packaged baked goods like muffins and pastries often contain refined flours, added sugars, and unhealthy fats like hydrogenated oils or butter. While they may provide some fiber from whole grain flours, the overall nutritional profile of these products can contribute to higher cholesterol levels when consumed in excess.

3. **Certain Ready-to-Eat Cereals:**

   - Explanation: Some ready-to-eat cereals marketed as healthy options may contain added sugars, artificial flavors, and partially hydrogenated oils. While they may provide some fiber from whole grains like wheat or oats, the added sugars and unhealthy fats can offset the potential cholesterol-lowering benefits of the fiber.

4. **Sweetened Flavored Yogurts:**

   - Explanation: Flavored yogurts often contain added sugars, artificial flavors, and sometimes unhealthy fats like palm oil or coconut oil. While yogurt itself can be a good source of protein and calcium, the added sugars and fats in flavored varieties can contribute to higher cholesterol levels, particularly when consumed regularly.

5. **Certain Packaged Bread Products:**

   - Explanation: Some packaged bread products, such as white bread or sweetened breads, may contain refined flours, added sugars, and unhealthy fats. While whole grain bread is generally a better choice for heart health, certain packaged bread products may contain additives that could contribute to higher cholesterol levels.

It's important to read food labels carefully and choose whole grain and fiber-rich foods that are minimally processed and free from added sugars, unhealthy fats, and artificial additives. Incorporating a variety of whole grains, fruits, vegetables, lean proteins, and healthy fats into your diet can help support heart health and maintain healthy cholesterol levels.

Chapter 7
Low Cholesterol Breakfast

Fruit Salad with Honey-Lime Dressing

Servings: 4

Preparation Time: 15 minutes

Ingredients:

- 2 cups mixed fresh fruits (strawberries, blueberries, kiwi, pineapple)

- 2 tablespoons honey

- 1 tablespoon fresh lime juice

- 1 teaspoon lime zest

- Fresh mint leaves for garnish

Instructions:

1. Wash and prepare the fruits. Cut them into bite-sized pieces and place them in a large mixing bowl.

2. In a small bowl, whisk together honey, lime juice, and lime zest.

3. Pour the honey-lime dressing over the fruits and gently toss to coat evenly.

4. Transfer the fruit salad to a serving bowl or individual dishes.

5. Garnish with fresh mint leaves.

Nutritional Information: Calories: 90 | Fat: 0g | Cholesterol: 0mg | Sodium: 0mg | Protein: 1g | Carbohydrates: 24g | Fiber: 3g

Greek Yogurt Parfait with Berries

Servings: 2

Preparation Time: 10 minutes

Ingredients:

- 1 cup non-fat Greek yogurt

- 1 cup mixed berries (strawberries, raspberries, blueberries)

- 2 tablespoons honey

- 2 tablespoons chopped nuts (almonds, walnuts)

- Fresh mint leaves for garnish (optional)

Instructions:

1. In serving glasses or bowls, layer Greek yogurt, mixed berries, and chopped nuts.

2. Drizzle honey over the top of each parfait.

3. Garnish with fresh mint leaves if desired.

Nutritional Information: Calories: 170 | Fat: 5g | Cholesterol: 0mg | Sodium: 35mg | Protein: 14g | Carbohydrates: 20g | Fiber: 4g

Helpful Tips: For added crunch and nutrition, use granola instead of nuts. This parfait is not only low in cholesterol but also a good source of protein.

Chia Seed Pudding

Servings: 2

Preparation Time: 5 minutes, plus chilling time

Ingredients:

- 1/4 cup chia seeds

- 1 cup unsweetened almond milk

- 1 tablespoon honey or maple syrup

- 1/2 teaspoon vanilla extract

- Fresh berries for topping

Instructions:

1. In a bowl, mix together chia seeds, almond milk, honey (or maple syrup), and vanilla extract.

2. Cover and refrigerate for at least 2 hours, or overnight, until the mixture thickens and has a pudding-like consistency.

3. Stir well before serving and top with fresh berries.

Nutritional Information: Calories: 110 | Fat: 5g | Cholesterol: 0mg | Sodium: 80mg | Protein: 4g | Carbohydrates: 14g | Fiber: 7g

Helpful Tips: Experiment with different flavors by adding cocoa powder or cinnamon to the pudding mixture before refrigerating.

Banana Oat Pancakes

Servings: 2

Preparation Time: 15 minutes

Ingredients:

- 1 ripe banana
- 1/2 cup rolled oats
- 2 eggs
- 1/2 teaspoon vanilla extract
- 1/2 teaspoon ground cinnamon
- 1/4 teaspoon baking powder
- Maple syrup and fresh berries for serving

Instructions:

1. In a blender, combine banana, rolled oats, eggs, vanilla extract, cinnamon, and baking powder. Blend until smooth.

2. Heat a non-stick skillet over medium heat and lightly grease with cooking spray or oil.

3. Pour 1/4 cup of batter onto the skillet for each pancake.

4. Cook for 2-3 minutes, or until bubbles form on the surface. Flip and cook for an additional 1-2 minutes, until golden brown.

5. Repeat with the remaining batter.

6. Serve warm with maple syrup and fresh berries.

Nutritional Information: Calories: 240 | Fat: 7g | Cholesterol: 185mg | Sodium: 80mg | Protein: 10g | Carbohydrates: 35g | Fiber: 4g

Berry Smoothie Bowl

Servings: 2

Preparation Time: 10 minutes

Ingredients:

- 1 cup mixed berries (strawberries, blueberries, raspberries)

- 1 frozen banana

- 1/2 cup unsweetened almond milk

- 1 tablespoon honey or maple syrup

- Toppings: sliced fresh fruits, shredded coconut, chia seeds, granola

Instructions:

1. In a blender, combine mixed berries, frozen banana, almond milk, and honey (or maple syrup). Blend until smooth and creamy.

2. Pour the smoothie into bowls.

3. Top with sliced fresh fruits, shredded coconut, chia seeds, and granola.

Nutritional Information: Calories: 150 | Fat: 2g | Cholesterol: 0mg | Sodium: 60mg | Protein: 2g | Carbohydrates: 35g | Fiber: 7g

Helpful Tips: Use frozen berries to make the smoothie thicker and colder. Customize your toppings according to your preference.

Egg White Omelette with Spinach and Tomatoes

Servings: 1

Preparation Time: 10 minutes

Ingredients:

- 3 egg whites
- 1/2 cup fresh spinach leaves
- 1/4 cup cherry tomatoes, halved

Instructions:

1. Heat a non-stick skillet over medium heat and lightly coat with cooking spray.
2. In a bowl, whisk together egg whites, salt, and pepper.
3. Pour the egg mixture into the skillet.
4. Cook for 2-3 minutes, or until the edges start to set.
5. Add spinach leaves and cherry tomatoes on one half of the omelette.
6. Carefully fold the other half of the omelette over the filling.
7. Cook for an additional 1-2 minutes, or until the omelette is cooked through.
8. Slide the omelette onto a plate and serve.

Nutritional Information: Calories: 70 | Fat: 0g | Cholesterol: 0mg | Sodium: 260mg | Protein: 15g | Carbohydrates: 4g | Fiber: 1g

Helpful Tips: Use a non-stick skillet and avoid overcooking the omelette to keep it fluffy and tender. You can add other vegetables like mushrooms or bell peppers.

Apple Cinnamon Baked Oatmeal

Servings: 4

Preparation Time: 40 minutes

Ingredients:

- 2 cups rolled oats
- 1 apple, peeled and diced
- 2 cups unsweetened almond milk
- 1/4 cup maple syrup
- 1 teaspoon ground cinnamon
- 1/4 teaspoon salt
- 1/4 cup chopped nuts (walnuts, almonds)

Instructions:

1. Preheat oven to 375°F (190°C). Grease a baking dish with cooking spray or oil.
2. In a large bowl, mix together rolled oats, diced apple, almond milk, maple syrup, cinnamon, and salt.
3. Pour the mixture into the prepared baking dish.
4. Sprinkle chopped nuts on top.
5. Bake for 30 minutes, or until the top is golden brown and the oats are set.
6. Remove from the oven and let it cool for a few minutes before serving.
7. Serve warm with fresh berries.

Nutritional Information: Calories: 250 | Fat: 8g | Cholesterol: 0mg | Sodium: 140mg | Protein: 7g | Carbohydrates: 40g | Fiber: 6g

Strawberry Banana Smoothie

Servings: 2

Preparation Time: 5 minutes

Ingredients:

- 1 cup frozen strawberries
- 1 ripe banana
- 1 cup unsweetened almond milk
- 1 tablespoon honey or maple syrup
- Ice cubes (optional)

Instructions:

1. In a blender, combine frozen strawberries, banana, almond milk, and honey (or maple syrup).
2. Add ice cubes if you prefer a thicker smoothie.
3. Blend until smooth and creamy.
4. Pour into glasses and serve immediately.

Nutritional Information: Calories: 120 | Fat: 1g | Cholesterol: 0mg | Sodium: 80mg | Protein: 2g | Carbohydrates: 30g | Fiber: 5g

Helpful Tips: You can add a tablespoon of chia seeds or ground flaxseeds for extra fiber and omega-3 fatty acids.

Veggie Breakfast Hash

Servings: 2

Preparation Time: 20 minutes

Ingredients:

- 2 medium potatoes, peeled and diced
- 1/2 onion, diced
- 1 bell pepper, diced
- 1/2 zucchini, diced
- 2 cloves garlic, minced
- 1 teaspoon paprika

Instructions:

1. Place diced potatoes in a microwave-safe bowl and microwave for 3-4 minutes, or until slightly tender.
2. Heat a non-stick skillet over medium heat and lightly coat with cooking spray.
3. Add diced onion, bell pepper, and zucchini to the skillet. Sauté for 3-4 minutes, or until softened.
4. Add minced garlic, paprika, salt, and pepper. Cook for an additional 1 minute.
5. Stir in the microwaved potatoes and cook for 5-7 minutes, or until the potatoes are golden brown and cooked through.
6. Remove from heat and garnish with fresh parsley before serving.

Nutritional Information: Calories: 180 | Fat: 0g | Cholesterol: 0mg | Sodium: 40mg | Protein: 4g | Carbohydrates: 40g | Fiber: 5g

Mango Banana Smoothie Bowl

Servings: 2

Preparation Time: 10 minutes

Ingredients:

- 1 ripe mango, peeled and diced

- 1 ripe banana

- 1/2 cup unsweetened almond milk

- 1 tablespoon honey or maple syrup

- Toppings: sliced fresh fruits, shredded coconut, chia seeds, granola

Instructions:

1. In a blender, combine diced mango, banana, almond milk, and honey (or maple syrup).

2. Blend until smooth and creamy.

3. Pour the smoothie into bowls.

4. Top with sliced fresh fruits, shredded coconut, chia seeds, and granola.

Nutritional Information: Calories: 180 | Fat: 1g | Cholesterol: 0mg | Sodium: 60mg | Protein: 2g | Carbohydrates: 40g | Fiber: 5g

Helpful Tips: Adjust the thickness of the smoothie by adding more or less almond milk. You can also use frozen mango for a colder smoothie bowl.

Chapter 8
Low Cholesterol Main Courses

Grilled Lemon Herb Chicken Breast

Servings: 4

Cooking Time: 25 minutes

Ingredients:

- 4 boneless, skinless chicken breasts

- 2 tablespoons olive oil

- 2 tablespoons fresh lemon juice

- 2 cloves garlic, minced.

- 1 teaspoon dried oregano

- 1 teaspoon dried thyme

- Salt and pepper to taste

- Lemon slices and fresh herbs for garnish

Instructions:

1. In a small bowl, whisk together olive oil, lemon juice, minced garlic, oregano, thyme, salt, and pepper.

2. Place chicken breasts in a resealable plastic bag and pour the marinade over them. Seal the bag and massage the marinade into the chicken. Marinate in the refrigerator for at least 30 minutes.

3. Preheat grill to medium-high heat.

4. Remove chicken from the marinade and discard the excess marinade.

5. Grill chicken for 6-7 minutes on each side, or until no longer pink in the center and the juices run clear.

6. Remove from the grill and let it rest for a few minutes before serving.

7. Garnish with lemon slices and fresh herbs.

Nutritional Information: Calories: 220 | Fat: 9g | Cholesterol: 80mg | Sodium: 280mg | Protein: 29g | Carbohydrates: 2g | Fiber: 0g

Helpful Tips: Marinating the chicken for a longer time will enhance the flavor. Be careful not to overcook to keep the chicken juicy.

Baked Lemon Garlic Salmon

Servings: 4

Cooking Time: 20 minutes

Ingredients:

- 4 salmon fillets

- 2 tablespoons olive oil

- 2 cloves garlic, minced.

- 2 tablespoons fresh lemon juice

- 1 teaspoon lemon zest

- 1 teaspoon dried oregano

- Salt and pepper to taste

- Lemon slices for garnish

- Fresh parsley, chopped, for garnish

Instructions:

1. Preheat oven to 375°F (190°C).

2. In a small bowl, whisk together olive oil, minced garlic, lemon juice, lemon zest, oregano, salt, and pepper.

3. Place salmon fillets on a baking sheet lined with parchment paper.

4. Brush the salmon fillets with the prepared lemon garlic mixture.

5. Bake in the preheated oven for 12-15 minutes, or until the salmon is cooked through and flakes easily with a fork.

6. Remove from the oven and let it rest for a few minutes before serving.

7. Garnish with lemon slices and chopped parsley.

Nutritional Information: Calories: 280 | Fat: 17g | Cholesterol: 80mg | Sodium: 90mg | Protein: 30g | Carbohydrates: 2g | Fiber: 0g

Helpful Tips: Avoid overcooking the salmon to maintain its tenderness and juiciness.

Grilled Balsamic Chicken with Vegetables

Servings: 4

Cooking Time: 30 minutes

Ingredients:

- 4 boneless, skinless chicken breasts

- 2 tablespoons olive oil

- 3 tablespoons balsamic vinegar

- 2 cloves garlic, minced

- 1 teaspoon dried oregano

- 1 teaspoon dried basil

- Salt and pepper to taste

- 2 cups mixed vegetables (bell peppers, zucchini, cherry tomatoes)

- Fresh basil leaves for garnish

Instructions:

1. In a small bowl, whisk together olive oil, balsamic vinegar, minced garlic, oregano, basil, salt, and pepper.

2. Place chicken breasts in a resealable plastic bag and pour the marinade over them. Seal the bag and massage the marinade into the chicken. Marinate in the refrigerator for at least 30 minutes.

3. Preheat grill to medium-high heat.

4. Thread marinated chicken and mixed vegetables onto skewers.

5. Grill skewers for 6-7 minutes on each side, or until chicken is no longer pink in the center and vegetables are tender.

6. Remove from the grill and let it rest for a few minutes before serving.

7. Garnish with fresh basil leaves.

Nutritional Information: Calories: 250 | Fat: 10g | Cholesterol: 80mg | Sodium: 120mg | Protein: 30g | Carbohydrates: 8g | Fiber: 2g

Helpful Tips: Soak wooden skewers in water for 30 minutes before grilling to prevent them from burning.

Honey Garlic Shrimp Stir Fry

Servings: 4

Cooking Time: 20 minutes

Ingredients:

- 1 lb (450g) large shrimp, peeled and deveined

- 2 tablespoons olive oil

- 3 cloves garlic, minced

- 2 tablespoons honey

- 2 tablespoons soy sauce

- 1 tablespoon freshly grated ginger

- 1 teaspoon sesame oil

- 2 cups mixed vegetables (broccoli, bell peppers, snap peas)

- Sesame seeds and chopped green onions for garnish

Instructions:

1. In a small bowl, whisk together honey, soy sauce, and sesame oil. Set aside.

2. Heat olive oil in a large pan or wok over medium-high heat.

3. Add minced garlic and grated ginger, and sauté for 1 minute.

4. Add shrimp to the pan and cook until pink, about 2-3 minutes.

5. Stir in the mixed vegetables and cook until they are tender-crisp, about 3-4 minutes.

6. Pour the honey garlic sauce over the shrimp and vegetables. Stir until everything is well coated and the sauce has thickened slightly.

7. Remove from heat and garnish with sesame seeds and chopped green onions.

Nutritional Information: Calories: 200 | Fat: 8g | Cholesterol: 150mg | Sodium: 480mg | Protein: 25g | Carbohydrates: 14g | Fiber: 2g

Helpful Tips: Do not overcook the shrimp to keep them tender and juicy.

Lemon Garlic Tilapia

Servings: 4

Cooking Time: 15 minutes

Ingredients:

- 4 tilapia fillets

- 2 tablespoons olive oil

- 2 cloves garlic, minced

- 2 tablespoons fresh lemon juice

- 1 teaspoon lemon zest

- 1 teaspoon dried parsley

- Salt and pepper to taste

- Lemon slices for garnish

Instructions:

1. In a small bowl, whisk together olive oil, minced garlic, lemon juice, lemon zest, parsley, salt, and pepper.

2. Preheat oven to 400°F (200°C).

3. Place tilapia fillets on a baking sheet lined with parchment paper.

4. Brush the tilapia fillets with the prepared lemon garlic mixture.

5. Bake in the preheated oven for 10-12 minutes, or until the fish is cooked through and flakes easily with a fork.

6. Remove from the oven and let it rest for a few minutes before serving.

7. Garnish with lemon slices.

Nutritional Information: Calories: 160 | Fat: 8g | Cholesterol: 40mg | Sodium: 120mg | Protein: 21g | Carbohydrates: 2g | Fiber: 0g

Helpful Tips: Check for doneness after 10 minutes to avoid overcooking the tilapia.

Vegetable Stir Fry with Tofu

Servings: 4

Cooking Time: 20 minutes

Ingredients:

- 1 block (14 oz) extra firm tofu, pressed and cubed

- 2 tablespoons sesame oil

- 3 cloves garlic, minced

- 1 tablespoon freshly grated ginger

- 2 cups mixed vegetables (bell peppers, broccoli, carrots, snap peas)

- 3 tablespoons low-sodium soy sauce

- 1 tablespoon rice vinegar

- 1 teaspoon honey

- Sesame seeds and sliced green onions for garnish

Instructions:

1. Heat sesame oil in a large pan or wok over medium-high heat.

2. Add minced garlic and grated ginger, and sauté for 1 minute.

3. Add cubed tofu to the pan and cook until golden brown, about 5-6 minutes. Remove tofu from the pan and set aside.

4. In the same pan, add a little more sesame oil if needed and stir-fry mixed vegetables until they are tender-crisp, about 3-4 minutes.

5. In a small bowl, whisk together soy sauce, rice vinegar, and honey.

6. Return the tofu to the pan, then pour the sauce over the tofu and vegetables. Stir until everything is well coated and the sauce has thickened slightly.

7. Remove from heat and garnish with sesame seeds and sliced green onions.

Nutritional Information: Calories: 220 | Fat: 12g | Cholesterol: 0mg | Sodium: 350mg | Protein: 14g | Carbohydrates: 15g | Fiber: 4g

Helpful Tips: Use firm or extra firm tofu for stir-frying to prevent it from falling apart.

Quinoa Stuffed Bell Peppers

Servings: 4

Cooking Time: 40 minutes

Ingredients:

- 4 bell peppers, tops removed and seeded

- 1 cup quinoa, cooked

- 1 can (15 oz) black beans, drained and rinsed

- 1 cup corn kernels

- 1 cup cherry tomatoes, halved

- 1 teaspoon cumin

- 1 teaspoon chili powder

- Salt and pepper to taste

- Fresh cilantro, chopped, for garnish

Instructions:

1. Preheat oven to 375°F (190°C).

2. In a large bowl, combine cooked quinoa, black beans, corn kernels, cherry tomatoes, cumin, chili powder, salt, and pepper.

3. Spoon the quinoa mixture into each bell pepper until they are full.

4. Place stuffed bell peppers in a baking dish.

5. Cover the dish with foil and bake in the preheated oven for 25-30 minutes, or until the peppers are tender.

6. Remove from the oven and let it cool for a few minutes before serving.

7. Garnish with chopped fresh cilantro.

Nutritional Information: Calories: 300 | Fat: 2g | Cholesterol: 0mg | Sodium: 280mg | Protein: 12g | Carbohydrates: 60g | Fiber: 12g

Helpful Tips: You can add some shredded low-fat cheese on top of the stuffed peppers during the last 5 minutes of baking, if desired.

Lentil Vegetable Soup

Servings: 6

Cooking Time: 45 minutes

Ingredients:

- 1 cup green lentils, rinsed and drained

- 1 tablespoon olive oil

- 1 onion, diced

- 3 cloves garlic, minced

- 2 carrots, diced

- 2 stalks celery, diced

- 1 can (14.5 oz) diced tomatoes

- 6 cups low-sodium vegetable broth

- 1 teaspoon dried thyme

- 1 teaspoon dried oregano

- Salt and pepper to taste

- Fresh parsley, chopped, for garnish

Instructions:

1. Heat olive oil in a large pot over medium heat.

2. Add diced onion and sauté until translucent, about 3-4 minutes.

3. Add minced garlic, diced carrots, and diced celery. Sauté for an additional 3-4 minutes.

4. Add rinsed green lentils, diced tomatoes, vegetable broth, dried thyme, dried oregano, salt, and pepper to the pot. Stir to combine.

5. Bring the soup to a boil, then reduce the heat to low and let it simmer for 30-35 minutes, or until the lentils are tender.

6. Taste and adjust seasoning if needed.

7. Remove from heat and garnish with chopped fresh parsley before serving.

Nutritional Information: Calories: 220 | Fat: 4g | Cholesterol: 0mg | Sodium: 480mg | Protein: 13g | Carbohydrates: 35g | Fiber: 14g

Helpful Tips: You can add spinach or kale to the soup during the last 5 minutes of cooking for added nutrition.

Turkey and Vegetable Skillet

Servings: 4

Cooking Time: 25 minutes

Ingredients:

- 1 lb (450g) ground turkey

- 2 tablespoons olive oil

- 1 onion, diced

- 2 cloves garlic, minced

- 2 cups mixed vegetables (bell peppers, zucchini, carrots)

- 1 teaspoon dried oregano

- 1 teaspoon paprika

- Salt and pepper to taste

- Fresh parsley, chopped, for garnish

Instructions:

1. Heat olive oil in a large skillet over medium heat.

2. Add diced onion and sauté until translucent, about 3-4 minutes.

3. Add minced garlic and ground turkey to the skillet. Cook until the turkey is browned, breaking it up with a spoon, about 5-6 minutes.

4. Add mixed vegetables, dried oregano, paprika, salt, and pepper to the skillet. Cook for an additional 5-7 minutes, or until the vegetables are tender.

5. Taste and adjust seasoning if needed.

6. Remove from heat and garnish with chopped fresh parsley before serving.

Nutritional Information: Calories: 260 | Fat: 14g | Cholesterol: 60mg | Sodium: 100mg | Protein: 25g | Carbohydrates: 10g | Fiber: 3g

Helpful Tips: You can serve this turkey and vegetable skillet over brown rice or quinoa for a heartier meal.

Lemon Herb Baked Cod

Servings: 4

Cooking Time: 20 minutes

Ingredients:

- 4 cod fillets

- 2 tablespoons olive oil

- 2 tablespoons fresh lemon juice

- 2 cloves garlic, minced

- 1 teaspoon dried thyme

- 1 teaspoon dried parsley

- Salt and pepper to taste

- Lemon slices for garnish

Instructions:

1. Preheat oven to 400°F (200°C).

2. In a small bowl, whisk together olive oil, lemon juice, minced garlic, thyme, parsley, salt, and pepper.

3. Place cod fillets on a baking sheet lined with parchment paper.

4. Brush the cod fillets with the prepared lemon herb mixture.

5. Bake in the preheated oven for 12-15 minutes, or until the fish is cooked through and flakes easily with a fork.

6. Remove from the oven and let it rest for a few minutes before serving.

7. Garnish with lemon slices.

Nutritional Information: Calories: 180 | Fat: 8g | Cholesterol: 55mg | Sodium: 220mg | Protein: 23g | Carbohydrates: 2g | Fiber: 0g

Helpful Tips: Choose wild-caught cod for a healthier option. Adjust the baking time depending on the thickness of the cod fillets.

Slow Cooker Vegetable Curry

Servings: 6

Cooking Time: 4 hours on high or 8 hours on low

Ingredients:

- 2 large potatoes, peeled and diced

- 3 carrots, sliced

- 1 large onion, chopped

- 1 red bell pepper, chopped

- 1 green bell pepper, chopped

- 1 cup cauliflower florets

- 1 cup green beans, trimmed and halved

- 2 cloves garlic, minced

- 1 can (14 oz) diced tomatoes, undrained

- 1 can (14 oz) coconut milk (light)

- 2 tablespoons curry powder

- 1 teaspoon ground turmeric

- 1 teaspoon ground cumin

- 1/2 teaspoon ground ginger

- Salt and pepper to taste

- Fresh cilantro, chopped (for garnish)

- Cooked rice (optional, for serving)

Instructions:

1. Place potatoes, carrots, onion, bell peppers, cauliflower, green beans, and garlic in the slow cooker.

2. In a medium bowl, mix together diced tomatoes, coconut milk, curry powder, turmeric, cumin, ginger, salt, and pepper.

3. Pour the mixture over the vegetables in the slow cooker.

4. Stir until the vegetables are evenly coated with the sauce.

5. Cover and cook on high for 4 hours or low for 8 hours, until the vegetables are tender.

6. Serve hot over cooked rice, if desired, and garnish with fresh cilantro.

Nutritional Information: Calories: 180 | Fat: 10g | Cholesterol: 0mg | Sodium: 280mg | Protein: 3g | Carbohydrates: 21g | Fiber: 5g

Helpful Tips: Add the coconut milk near the end of the cooking time to prevent curdling. Adjust the curry powder to suit your taste preferences.

Slow Cooker Lentil Soup

Servings: 6

Cooking Time: 6-8 hours on low

Ingredients:

- 1 cup dry lentils, rinsed and drained

- 3 carrots, diced

- 2 stalks celery, diced

- 1 onion, chopped

- 2 cloves garlic, minced

- 1 can (14 oz) diced tomatoes, undrained

- 6 cups vegetable broth

- 1 teaspoon dried thyme

- 1 teaspoon dried oregano

- 1 teaspoon ground cumin

- Salt and pepper to taste

- Fresh parsley, chopped (for garnish)

Instructions:

1. In the slow cooker, combine lentils, carrots, celery, onion, garlic, diced tomatoes, vegetable broth, thyme, oregano, cumin, salt, and pepper.

2. Stir well to combine.

3. Cover and cook on low for 6-8 hours, until the lentils and vegetables are tender.

4. Before serving, taste and adjust seasoning if needed.

5. Ladle into bowls and garnish with fresh parsley.

Nutritional Information: Calories: 180 | Fat: 1g | Cholesterol: 0mg | Sodium: 650mg | Protein: 12g | Carbohydrates: 33g | Fiber: 15g

Helpful Tips: For a thicker soup, blend a portion of the soup with an immersion blender and return it to the slow cooker before serving.

Slow Cooker Ratatouille

Servings: 6

Cooking Time: 6 hours on low

Ingredients:

- 1 eggplant, diced

- 2 zucchinis, sliced

- 1 onion, diced

- 1 red bell pepper, chopped

- 1 yellow bell pepper, chopped

- 3 cloves garlic, minced

- 1 can (14 oz) diced tomatoes, undrained

- 2 tablespoons tomato paste

- 1 teaspoon dried thyme

- 1 teaspoon dried oregano

- 1/2 teaspoon dried basil

- Salt and pepper to taste

- Fresh basil, chopped (for garnish)

Instructions:

1. In the slow cooker, combine eggplant, zucchinis, onion, bell peppers, garlic, diced tomatoes, tomato paste, thyme, oregano, basil, salt, and pepper.

2. Stir well to combine.

3. Cover and cook on low for 6 hours, until the vegetables are tender.

4. Before serving, taste and adjust seasoning if needed.

5. Ladle into bowls and garnish with fresh basil.

Nutritional Information: Calories: 70 | Fat: 0g | Cholesterol: 0mg | Sodium: 330mg | Protein: 3g | Carbohydrates: 16g | Fiber: 6g

Helpful Tips: For added depth of flavor, sauté the onions and garlic before adding them to the slow cooker. Ratatouille can be served hot, cold, or at room temperature.

Slow Cooker Butternut Squash Soup

Servings: 6

Cooking Time: 4 hours on high or 6-8 hours on low

Ingredients:

- 1 medium butternut squash, peeled, seeded, and diced
- 2 carrots, chopped
- 1 apple, peeled, cored, and chopped
- 1 onion, chopped
- 2 cloves garlic, minced
- 4 cups vegetable broth
- 1 teaspoon ground cinnamon
- 1/2 teaspoon ground nutmeg
- Salt and pepper to taste
- 1/2 cup coconut milk (light), for garnish
- Fresh chives, chopped (for garnish)

Instructions:

1. In the slow cooker, combine butternut squash, carrots, apple, onion, garlic, vegetable broth, cinnamon, nutmeg, salt, and pepper.
2. Stir well to combine.
3. Cover and cook on high for 4 hours or low for 6-8 hours, until the vegetables are tender.

4.   Use an immersion blender to blend the soup until smooth.

5.   Taste and adjust seasoning if needed.

6.   Serve hot, garnished with a drizzle of coconut milk and fresh chives.

Nutritional Information: Calories: 90 | Fat: 1g | Cholesterol: 0mg | Sodium: 650mg | Protein: 2g | Carbohydrates: 20g | Fiber: 4g

Helpful Tips: To easily peel the butternut squash, pierce it with a fork and microwave it for 2-3 minutes to soften the skin. Allow it to cool slightly before peeling and dicing. Adjust the consistency of the soup by adding more vegetable broth if desired.

Chapter 9
Low Cholesterol Soups & Salads

Cucumber and Tomato Salad

Servings: 4
Preparation Time: 10 minutes

Ingredients:

- 2 large cucumbers, sliced
- 2 large tomatoes, diced
- 1/4 red onion, thinly sliced
- 2 tablespoons fresh lemon juice
- 1 tablespoon olive oil
- 1 tablespoon chopped fresh parsley

Instructions:

1. In a large bowl, combine sliced cucumbers, diced tomatoes, and thinly sliced red onion.
2. Drizzle with fresh lemon juice and olive oil.
3. Add chopped parsley, salt, and pepper.
4. Toss gently to combine.
5. Serve chilled.

Nutritional Information: Calories: 45 | Fat: 3g | Cholesterol: 0mg | Sodium: 5mg | Protein: 1g | Carbohydrates: 5g | Fiber: 1g

Helpful Tips: For the best flavor, allow the salad to sit for 15-20 minutes before serving to let the flavors meld together.

Gazpacho (Chilled Tomato Soup)

Servings: 4

Preparation Time: 15 minutes, plus chilling time

Ingredients:

- 6 ripe tomatoes, chopped
- 1 cucumber, peeled and chopped
- 1 red bell pepper, seeded and chopped
- 1/4 red onion, chopped
- 2 cloves garlic, minced
- 2 tablespoons olive oil
- 3 tablespoons red wine vinegar
- 1 teaspoon Worcestershire sauce (optional)

Instructions:

1. In a blender or food processor, combine chopped tomatoes, cucumber, red bell pepper, red onion, and minced garlic.
2. Blend until smooth.
3. Add olive oil, red wine vinegar, Worcestershire sauce (if using), salt, and pepper. Blend until well combined.
4. Transfer the mixture to a large bowl, cover, and refrigerate for at least 1 hour.
5. Serve chilled, garnished with fresh basil leaves.

Nutritional Information: Calories: 80 | Fat: 5g | Cholesterol: 0mg | Sodium: 150mg | Protein: 2g | Carbohydrates: 9g | Fiber: 2g

Helpful Tips: Adjust the consistency by adding a little water if the soup is too thick. You can also make it spicy by adding a dash of hot sauce.

Caprese Salad

Servings: 4

Preparation Time: 10 minutes

Ingredients:

- 2 large tomatoes, sliced

- 1 ball fresh mozzarella cheese, sliced

- Fresh basil leaves

- 2 tablespoons balsamic vinegar

- 1 tablespoon olive oil

Instructions:

1. Arrange tomato slices and mozzarella slices on a serving platter, alternating and overlapping them.

2. Tuck fresh basil leaves between the tomato and mozzarella slices.

3. Drizzle with balsamic vinegar and olive oil.

4. Season with salt and pepper.

5. Serve immediately.

Nutritional Information: Calories: 150 | Fat: 10g | Cholesterol: 20mg | Sodium: 300mg | Protein: 7g | Carbohydrates: 8g | Fiber: 1g

Helpful Tips: Use ripe, in-season tomatoes and fresh mozzarella for the best flavor. You can also sprinkle with a pinch of dried oregano or fresh ground black pepper.

Cucumber and Dill Salad

Servings: 4

Preparation Time: 10 minutes

Ingredients:

- 2 large cucumbers, thinly sliced
- 1/4 red onion, thinly sliced
- 1/4 cup chopped fresh dill
- 2 tablespoons white vinegar
- 1 tablespoon olive oil
- 1 teaspoon sugar (optional)

Instructions:

1. In a large bowl, combine thinly sliced cucumbers, thinly sliced red onion, and chopped fresh dill.

2. In a small bowl, whisk together white vinegar, olive oil, sugar (if using), salt, and pepper.

3. Pour the dressing over the cucumber mixture and toss gently to coat.

4. Serve immediately or refrigerate until ready to serve.

Nutritional Information: Calories: 45 | Fat: 3g | Cholesterol: 0mg | Sodium: 10mg | Protein: 1g | Carbohydrates: 5g | Fiber: 1g

Helpful Tips: For a stronger dill flavor, let the salad marinate in the refrigerator for at least 30 minutes before serving.

Watermelon Feta Salad

Servings: 4

Preparation Time: 15 minutes

Ingredients:

- 4 cups cubed watermelon

- 1/2 cup crumbled feta cheese

- 1/4 cup fresh mint leaves, chopped

- 2 tablespoons balsamic glaze

- 1 tablespoon olive oil

Instructions:

1. In a large bowl, combine cubed watermelon, crumbled feta cheese, and chopped fresh mint leaves.

2. Drizzle with balsamic glaze and olive oil.

3. Season with salt and pepper.

4. Toss gently to combine.

5. Serve chilled.

Nutritional Information: Calories: 120 | Fat: 6g | Cholesterol: 20mg | Sodium: 150mg | Protein: 3g | Carbohydrates: 15g | Fiber: 1g

Helpful Tips: Choose seedless watermelon for easier preparation. You can also add a handful of arugula to make it a bit heartier.

Spinach and Strawberry Salad

Servings: 4

Preparation Time: 10 minutes

Ingredients:

- 4 cups baby spinach leaves
- 1 cup sliced strawberries
- 1/4 cup sliced almonds
- 2 tablespoons balsamic vinegar
- 1 tablespoon olive oil
- 1 teaspoon honey

Instructions:

1. In a large bowl, combine baby spinach leaves, sliced strawberries, and sliced almonds.

2. In a small bowl, whisk together balsamic vinegar, olive oil, honey, salt, and pepper.

3. Drizzle the dressing over the salad and toss gently to combine.

4. Serve immediately.

Nutritional Information: Calories: 90 | Fat: 6g | Cholesterol: 0mg | Sodium: 50mg | Protein: 3g | Carbohydrates: 8g | Fiber: 3g

Helpful Tips: For a variation, you can add grilled chicken or shrimp to turn it into a complete meal.

Greek Salad

Servings: 4

Preparation Time: 15 minutes

Ingredients:

- 2 large tomatoes, chopped
- 1 cucumber, chopped
- 1/2 red onion, thinly sliced
- 1/2 cup Kalamata olives, pitted
- 1/2 cup crumbled feta cheese
- 2 tablespoons red wine vinegar
- 1 tablespoon olive oil
- 1 teaspoon dried oregano

Instructions:

1. In a large bowl, combine chopped tomatoes, chopped cucumber, thinly sliced red onion, Kalamata olives, and crumbled feta cheese.

2. In a small bowl, whisk together red wine vinegar, olive oil, dried oregano, salt, and pepper.

3. Drizzle the dressing over the salad and toss gently to combine.

4. Serve immediately.

Nutritional Information: Calories: 150 | Fat: 10g | Cholesterol: 20mg | Sodium: 400mg | Protein: 5g | Carbohydrates: 10g | Fiber: 3g

Helpful Tips: Serve with a side of whole-grain bread for a more filling meal.

Corn and Black Bean Salad

Servings: 4

Preparation Time: 15 minutes

Ingredients:

- 1 can (15 oz) black beans, drained and rinsed
- 1 cup corn kernels (fresh or canned)
- 1 red bell pepper, diced
- 1/4 cup red onion, finely chopped
- 1/4 cup fresh cilantro, chopped
- 2 tablespoons lime juice
- 1 tablespoon olive oil
- 1 teaspoon ground cumin

Instructions:

1. In a large bowl, combine black beans, corn kernels, diced red bell pepper, finely chopped red onion, and chopped fresh cilantro.
2. In a small bowl, whisk together lime juice, olive oil, ground cumin, salt, and pepper.
3. Drizzle the dressing over the salad and toss gently to combine.
4. Serve chilled.

Nutritional Information: Calories: 150 | Fat: 4g | Cholesterol: 0mg | Sodium: 300mg | Protein: 6g | Carbohydrates: 24g | Fiber: 6g

Helpful Tips: You can add diced avocado for extra creaminess. Make sure to use fresh lime juice for the best flavor.

Lentil Salad

Servings: 4

Preparation Time: 20 minutes

Ingredients:

- 1 cup cooked green lentils
- 1/2 cucumber, diced
- 1/2 red bell pepper, diced
- 1/4 red onion, finely chopped
- 2 tablespoons chopped fresh parsley
- 2 tablespoons lemon juice
- 1 tablespoon olive oil
- 1 teaspoon Dijon mustard

Instructions:

1. In a large bowl, combine cooked green lentils, diced cucumber, diced red bell pepper, finely chopped red onion, and chopped fresh parsley.
2. In a small bowl, whisk together lemon juice, olive oil, Dijon mustard, salt, and pepper.
3. Drizzle the dressing over the salad and toss gently to combine.
4. Serve chilled.

Nutritional Information: Calories: 120 | Fat: 4g | Cholesterol: 0mg | Sodium: 20mg | Protein: 5g | Carbohydrates: 17g | Fiber: 5g

Helpful Tips: You can add chopped cherry tomatoes for an extra burst of flavor and color.

Asian Cucumber Salad

Servings: 4

Preparation Time: 10 minutes

Ingredients:

- 2 large cucumbers, thinly sliced
- 1/4 cup rice vinegar
- 1 tablespoon soy sauce
- 1 tablespoon sesame oil
- 1 teaspoon honey
- 1/2 teaspoon red pepper flakes
- 1 tablespoon sesame seeds
- 2 green onions, thinly sliced

Instructions:

1. In a large bowl, combine thinly sliced cucumbers.
2. In a small bowl, whisk together rice vinegar, soy sauce, sesame oil, honey, and red pepper flakes.
3. Drizzle the dressing over the cucumbers and toss gently to combine.
4. Sprinkle sesame seeds and thinly sliced green onions on top.
5. Serve chilled.

Nutritional Information: Calories: 70 | Fat: 4g | Cholesterol: 0mg | Sodium: 160mg | Protein: 1g | Carbohydrates: 8g | Fiber: 1g

Helpful Tips: For an added crunch, you can sprinkle some crushed peanuts or cashews on top. Allow the salad to sit for a while before serving to let the flavors meld together.

Chapter 10

Low Cholesterol Snacks & Desserts

Mixed Berry Sorbet

Servings: 4

Preparation Time: 5 minutes, plus freezing time

Ingredients:

- 2 cups mixed berries (strawberries, blueberries, raspberries)

- 1/4 cup honey

- 2 tablespoons fresh lemon juice

Instructions:

1. Place the mixed berries, honey, and fresh lemon juice in a blender or food processor.

2. Blend until smooth.

3. Pour the mixture into a shallow dish.

4. Freeze for 3-4 hours, stirring every 30 minutes, until firm.

5. Serve the sorbet in chilled bowls.

Nutritional Information: Calories: 70 | Fat: 0g | Cholesterol: 0mg | Sodium: 0mg | Protein: 1g | Carbohydrates: 19g | Fiber: 3g

Helpful Tips: For a creamier texture, use an ice cream maker. If you don't have one, stirring the mixture while freezing will give it a smoother consistency.

Baked Cinnamon Apple Chips

Servings: 4

Preparation Time: 1 hour 30 minutes

Ingredients:

- 2 large apples, cored and thinly sliced

- 1 tablespoon granulated sugar

- 1 teaspoon ground cinnamon

Instructions:

1. Preheat the oven to 200°F (95°C). Line two baking sheets with parchment paper.

2. In a bowl, combine the granulated sugar and ground cinnamon.

3. Arrange the apple slices in a single layer on the prepared baking sheets.

4. Sprinkle the cinnamon-sugar mixture over the apple slices.

5. Bake for 1 hour, then flip the apple slices and bake for an additional 30 minutes, or until the chips are crisp.

6. Allow the apple chips to cool completely before serving.

Nutritional Information: Calories: 50 | Fat: 0g | Cholesterol: 0mg | Sodium: 0mg | Protein: 0g | Carbohydrates: 14g | Fiber: 2g

Helpful Tips: Store the apple chips in an airtight container to maintain crispness.

Chocolate-Dipped Strawberries

Servings: 4

Preparation Time: 20 minutes

Ingredients:

- 1 cup fresh strawberries, washed and dried

- 1/4 cup dark chocolate chips

Instructions:

1. Line a baking sheet with parchment paper.

2. In a microwave-safe bowl, melt the dark chocolate chips in the microwave in 30-second intervals, stirring until smooth.

3. Dip each strawberry into the melted chocolate, coating about two-thirds of the berry.

4. Place the dipped strawberries on the prepared baking sheet.

5. Allow the chocolate to set at room temperature for about 15 minutes, or place in the refrigerator for 5 minutes.

6. Serve the chocolate-dipped strawberries.

Nutritional Information: Calories: 45 | Fat: 2g | Cholesterol: 0mg | Sodium: 0mg | Protein: 1g | Carbohydrates: 7g | Fiber: 2g

Helpful Tips: For a festive touch, sprinkle crushed nuts or coconut flakes over the chocolate before it sets.

Lemon Sorbet

Servings: 4

Preparation Time: 5 minutes, plus freezing time

Ingredients:

- 1 cup water

- 1 cup fresh lemon juice

- 1/2 cup granulated sugar

- Zest of 1 lemon

Instructions:

1. In a saucepan, combine water, fresh lemon juice, granulated sugar, and lemon zest.

2. Heat over medium heat, stirring until the sugar is dissolved.

3. Remove from heat and let it cool to room temperature.

4. Pour the mixture into a shallow dish.

5. Freeze for 3-4 hours, stirring every 30 minutes, until firm.

6. Serve the sorbet in chilled bowls.

Nutritional Information: Calories: 80 | Fat: 0g | Cholesterol: 0mg | Sodium: 0mg | Protein: 0g | Carbohydrates: 21g | Fiber: 0g

Helpful Tips: For a tangier sorbet, increase the amount of lemon juice.

Baked Cinnamon Banana Chips

Servings: 4

Preparation Time: 2 hours

Ingredients:

- 2 ripe bananas

- 1 teaspoon ground cinnamon

Instructions:

1. Preheat the oven to 200°F (95°C). Line a baking sheet with parchment paper.

2. Peel the bananas and slice them into thin rounds.

3. Place the banana slices on the prepared baking sheet.

4. Sprinkle the ground cinnamon over the banana slices.

5. Bake for 1 hour, then flip the banana slices and bake for an additional 45-60 minutes, or until the chips are crisp.

6. Allow the banana chips to cool completely before serving.

Nutritional Information: Calories: 60 | Fat: 0g | Cholesterol: 0mg | Sodium: 0mg | Protein: 1g | Carbohydrates: 16g | Fiber: 2g

Helpful Tips: Keep an eye on the chips in the last 15 minutes to prevent burning.

Strawberry Frozen Yogurt Bark

Servings: 4

Preparation Time: 2 hours 10 minutes, plus freezing time

Ingredients:

- 2 cups plain Greek yogurt

- 1/4 cup honey

- 1 teaspoon vanilla extract

- 1 cup sliced strawberries

Instructions:

1. Line a baking sheet with parchment paper.

2. In a bowl, mix together Greek yogurt, honey, and vanilla extract until smooth.

3. Spread the yogurt mixture evenly onto the prepared baking sheet.

4. Sprinkle the sliced strawberries over the yogurt.

5. Place the baking sheet in the freezer and freeze for about 2 hours, or until firm.

6. Once frozen, break the bark into pieces and serve.

Nutritional Information: Calories: 100 | Fat: 0g | Cholesterol: 5mg | Sodium: 30mg | Protein: 7g | Carbohydrates: 20g | Fiber: 1g

Helpful Tips: You can use any combination of fruits for this recipe. Try blueberries, raspberries, or even mango.

Mango Sorbet

Servings: 4

Preparation Time: 5 minutes, plus freezing time

Ingredients:

- 2 ripe mangoes, peeled and chopped

- 1/4 cup honey

- 2 tablespoons fresh lime juice

Instructions:

1. Place the chopped mangoes, honey, and fresh lime juice in a blender or food processor.

2. Blend until smooth.

3. Pour the mixture into a shallow dish.

4. Freeze for 3-4 hours, stirring every 30 minutes, until firm.

5. Serve the sorbet in chilled bowls.

Nutritional Information: Calories: 100 | Fat: 0g | Cholesterol: 0mg | Sodium: 0mg | Protein: 1g | Carbohydrates: 27g | Fiber: 2g

Helpful Tips: For a creamier texture, use an ice cream maker. If you don't have one, stirring the mixture while freezing will give it a smoother consistency.

Frozen Grapes

Servings: 4

Preparation Time: 2 hours

Ingredients:

- 2 cups seedless grapes

Instructions:

1. Wash and pat dry the grapes.

2. Place the grapes in a single layer on a baking sheet lined with parchment paper.

3. Freeze for at least 2 hours until firm.

4. Serve the frozen grapes.

Nutritional Information: Calories: 60 | Fat: 0g | Cholesterol: 0mg | Sodium: 0mg | Protein: 1g | Carbohydrates: 16g | Fiber: 1g

Helpful Tips: You can also roll the grapes in flavored gelatin powder before freezing to add a fun twist.

Pineapple Sorbet

Servings: 4

Preparation Time: 5 minutes, plus freezing time

Ingredients:

- 2 cups fresh pineapple chunks

- 1/4 cup honey

- 2 tablespoons fresh lemon juice

Instructions:

1. Place the pineapple chunks, honey, and fresh lemon juice in a blender or food processor.

2. Blend until smooth.

3. Pour the mixture into a shallow dish.

4. Freeze for 3-4 hours, stirring every 30 minutes, until firm.

5. Serve the sorbet in chilled bowls.

Nutritional Information: Calories: 90 | Fat: 0g | Cholesterol: 0mg | Sodium: 0mg | Protein: 1g | Carbohydrates: 24g | Fiber: 1g

Helpful Tips: For a creamier texture, use an ice cream maker. If you don't have one, stirring the mixture while freezing will give it a smoother consistency.

Mixed Berry Smoothie Popsicles

Servings: 6

Preparation Time: 5 minutes, plus freezing time

Ingredients:

- 1 cup mixed berries (strawberries, blueberries, raspberries)

- 1 cup plain Greek yogurt

- 2 tablespoons honey

Instructions:

1. Place the mixed berries, Greek yogurt, and honey in a blender.

2. Blend until smooth.

3. Pour the mixture into popsicle molds.

4. Insert popsicle sticks and freeze for at least 4 hours, or until firm.

5. Once frozen, remove the popsicles from the molds and serve.

Nutritional Information: Calories: 60 | Fat: 0g | Cholesterol: 0mg | Sodium: 15mg | Protein: 3g | Carbohydrates: 12g | Fiber: 1g

Helpful Tips: Add a few whole berries to each popsicle mold for an extra burst of flavor and texture.

CONCLUSION

Congratulations on completing your journey through this comprehensive low cholesterol food list and cookbook! By incorporating these delicious and healthy recipes into your lifestyle, you've taken proactive steps toward a healthier heart and a happier life.

As you close this book, remember that the benefits of a low-cholesterol diet extend far beyond the delicious recipes. You will experience increased energy levels, improved mood, and enhanced overall well-being.

By embracing a low-cholesterol diet, you are not only nourishing your body but also nurturing your soul. Food is not just sustenance; it is an experience, a celebration of life, health, and happiness.

I encourage you to try out the recipes, share them with your loved ones, and most importantly, listen to your body. Pay attention to how these meals make you feel, both physically and emotionally. Your feedback is invaluable to me. I am always striving to improve and create content that best serves your needs.

Please take a moment to leave an honest review and share your thoughts. Your feedback will not only help me improve but will also guide and inspire others on their journey to better health.

Remember, this cookbook is just the beginning of your culinary adventure toward better health. Let's continue to explore, learn, and grow together. Together, we can achieve our health goals and lead happier, more fulfilling lives.

Thank you for allowing me to be a part of your health and wellness journey. Here's to a healthier, happier you!

BONUS 1
FOOD TRACKER

Food Item	Serving Size	Cholesterol (mg)
Oatmeal	1 cup cooked	0
Lentils	1 cup cooked	0
Quinoa	1 cup cooked	0
Almonds	1 oz	0
Avocado	1 medium	0
Olive Oil	1 tbsp	0
Broccoli	1 cup cooked	0
Spinach	1 cup cooked	0
Blueberries	1 cup	0
Strawberries	1 cup	0
Salmon	3 oz	55
Tofu	3 oz	0
Chicken Breast	3 oz	73
Turkey Breast	3 oz	46
Shrimp	3 oz	161
Tilapia	3 oz	56
Egg Whites	1 large	0
Skim Milk	1 cup	5
Greek Yogurt	1 cup	10
Brown Rice	1 cup cooked	0
Apples	1 medium	0

Oranges	1 medium	0
Carrots	1 cup	0
Celery	1 stalk	0
Garlic	1 clove	0
Onions	1 medium	0
Tomatoes	1 medium	0
Sweet Potatoes	1 medium	0
Green Tea	1 cup	0
Flaxseeds	1 tbsp	0
Chia Seeds	1 tbsp	0
Walnuts	1 oz	0
Pecans	1 oz	0
Brussels Sprouts	1 cup	0
Cucumber	1 cup	0
Zucchini	1 cup	0
Cauliflower	1 cup	0
Mushrooms	1 cup	0
Beets	1 cup	0
Asparagus	1 cup	0
Bell Peppers	1 medium	0
Eggplant	1 cup	0
Green Beans	1 cup	0
Peas	1 cup	0
Radishes	1 cup	0
Artichokes	1 medium	0
Cabbage	1 cup	0
Kiwi	1 medium	0

Pineapple	1 cup	0
Mango	1 medium	0
Papaya	1 cup	0
Grapes	1 cup	0
Pears	1 medium	0
Cranberries	1 cup	0
Peaches	1 medium	0
Cherries	1 cup	0
Blackberries	1 cup	0
Raspberries	1 cup	0
Plums	1 medium	0
Apricots	1 medium	0
Beets	1 cup	0
Pumpkin	1 cup	0
Butternut Squash	1 cup	0
Acorn Squash	1 cup	0
Spaghetti Squash	1 cup	0
Radicchio	1 cup	0
Turnips	1 cup	0
Watermelon	1 cup	0
Cantaloupe	1 cup	0
Honeydew Melon	1 cup	0
Cauliflower	1 cup	0
Green Peas	1 cup	0
Brussels Sprouts	1 cup	0
Fennel	1 cup	0
Leeks	1 cup	0

Okra	1 cup	0
Rutabaga	1 cup	0
Swiss Chard	1 cup	0
Tangerines	1 medium	0
Turnips	1 medium	0
Radishes	1 medium	0
Pomegranate	1 medium	0
Kohlrabi	1 cup	0
Arugula	1 cup	0
Starfruit	1 medium	0
Guava	1 medium	0
Lychee	1 cup	0
Passion Fruit	1 medium	0

BONUS 2
21 Day Meal Plan

Day	Breakfast	Lunch	Dinner
Day 1	Oatmeal with Blueberries (No added sugar)	Quinoa Salad with Spinach, Cherry Tomatoes, and Olive Oil Dressing	Baked Salmon with Steamed Broccoli
Day 2	Greek Yogurt with Sliced Almonds and Strawberries	Lentil Soup with Whole Grain Bread	Grilled Tofu with Stir-fried Vegetables
Day 3	Avocado Toast with Whole Grain Bread	Grilled Chicken Breast Salad with Balsamic Vinaigrette	Turkey Chili with Brown Rice
Day 4	Whole Grain Pancakes with Fresh Fruit	Tuna Salad on Whole Wheat Pita Bread	Baked Tilapia with Asparagus
Day 5	Scrambled Egg Whites with Sautéed Spinach and Tomatoes	Quinoa and Black Bean Wrap	Stir-fried Shrimp with Vegetables
Day 6	Smoothie with Kale, Banana, and Chia Seeds	Vegetable Stir-fry with Tofu	Grilled Chicken Breast with Steamed Green Beans
Day 7	Whole Grain Toast with Mashed Avocado	Lentil Salad with Mixed Greens and Lemon-Tahini Dressing	Baked Salmon with Roasted Brussels Sprouts

Day 8	Oatmeal with Sliced Banana and Walnuts	Turkey and Vegetable Soup	Baked Chicken with Cauliflower Rice
Day 9	Greek Yogurt with Honey and Mixed Berries	Grilled Tofu Salad with Balsamic Vinaigrette	Grilled Shrimp with Quinoa and Steamed Broccoli
Day 10	Whole Grain Waffles with Fresh Fruit	Chickpea Salad with Cucumber, Tomato, and Olive Oil Dressing	Baked Tilapia with Garlic Roasted Green Beans
Day 11	Smoothie Bowl with Spinach, Mango, and Flaxseeds	Turkey Wrap with Lettuce, Tomato, and Mustard	Grilled Chicken Breast with Steamed Carrots
Day 12	Avocado Toast with Sliced Tomato	Lentil and Vegetable Stir-fry	Baked Salmon with Grilled Asparagus
Day 13	Scrambled Egg Whites with Sautéed Spinach and Mushrooms	Quinoa Salad with Black Beans, Corn, and Lime Vinaigrette	Grilled Tofu with Stir-fried Vegetables
Day 14	Whole Grain Pancakes with Fresh Berries	Grilled Chicken Caesar Salad	Turkey Chili with Brown Rice
Day 15	Oatmeal with Blueberries (No added sugar)	Lentil Soup with Whole Grain Bread	Baked Tilapia with Steamed Broccoli
Day 16	Greek Yogurt with Sliced Almonds and Strawberries	Grilled Tofu Salad with Balsamic Vinaigrette	Stir-fried Shrimp with Vegetables

Day			
Day 17	Avocado Toast with Whole Grain Bread	Quinoa and Black Bean Wrap	Grilled Chicken Breast with Steamed Green Beans
Day 18	Whole Grain Waffles with Fresh Fruit	Tuna Salad on Whole Wheat Pita Bread	Baked Salmon with Asparagus
Day 19	Smoothie with Kale, Banana, and Chia Seeds	Chickpea Salad with Cucumber, Tomato, and Olive Oil Dressing	Baked Chicken with Cauliflower Rice
Day 20	Whole Grain Toast with Mashed Avocado	Grilled Tofu with Stir-fried Vegetables	Grilled Shrimp with Quinoa and Steamed Broccoli
Day 21	Scrambled Egg Whites with Sautéed Spinach and Tomatoes	Lentil Salad with Mixed Greens and Lemon-Tahini Dressing	Baked Chicken with Roasted Brussels Sprouts

MEAL PLANNER JOUNAL

Meal Planner Journal

Week of:

Monday	**Tuesday**	**Wednesday**
BREAKFAST	BREAKFAST	BREAKFAST
LUNCH	LUNCH	LUNCH
DINNER	DINNER	DINNER
SNACK	SNACK	SNACK
Thursday	**Friday**	**Saturday**
BREAKFAST	BREAKFAST	BREAKFAST
LUNCH	LUNCH	LUNCH
DINNER	DINNER	DINNER
SNACK	SNACK	SNACK
Sunday	NOTES	
BREAKFAST		
LUNCH		
DINNER		
SNACK		

Meal Planner Journal

Week of:

Monday	**Tuesday**	**Wednesday**
BREAKFAST	BREAKFAST	BREAKFAST
LUNCH	LUNCH	LUNCH
DINNER	DINNER	DINNER
SNACK	SNACK	SNACK

Thursday	**Friday**	**Saturday**
BREAKFAST	BREAKFAST	BREAKFAST
LUNCH	LUNCH	LUNCH
DINNER	DINNER	DINNER
SNACK	SNACK	SNACK

Sunday	NOTES:
BREAKFAST	
LUNCH	
DINNER	
SNACK	

Meal Planner Journal

Week of:

Monday

BREAKFAST

LUNCH

DINNER

SNACK

Tuesday

BREAKFAST

LUNCH

DINNER

SNACK

Wednesday

BREAKFAST

LUNCH

DINNER

SNACK

Thursday

BREAKFAST

LUNCH

DINNER

SNACK

Friday

BREAKFAST

LUNCH

DINNER

SNACK

Saturday

BREAKFAST

LUNCH

DINNER

SNACK

Sunday

BREAKFAST

LUNCH

DINNER

SNACK

NOTES:

Meal Planner Journal

Week of:

Monday	**Tuesday**	**Wednesday**

Monday

BREAKFAST

LUNCH

DINNER

SNACK

Tuesday

BREAKFAST

LUNCH

DINNER

SNACK

Wednesday

BREAKFAST

LUNCH

DINNER

SNACK

Thursday

BREAKFAST

LUNCH

DINNER

SNACK

Friday

BREAKFAST

LUNCH

DINNER

SNACK

Saturday

BREAKFAST

LUNCH

DINNER

SNACK

Sunday

BREAKFAST

LUNCH

DINNER

SNACK

NOTES:

Meal Planner Journal

Week of:

<table>
<tr><td>Monday</td><td>Tuesday</td><td>Wednesday</td></tr>
<tr><td>BREAKFAST

LUNCH

DINNER

SNACK</td><td>BREAKFAST

LUNCH

DINNER

SNACK</td><td>BREAKFAST

LUNCH

DINNER

SNACK</td></tr>
<tr><td>Thursday</td><td>Friday</td><td>Saturday</td></tr>
<tr><td>BREAKFAST

LUNCH

DINNER

SNACK</td><td>BREAKFAST

LUNCH

DINNER

SNACK</td><td>BREAKFAST

LUNCH

DINNER

SNACK</td></tr>
<tr><td>Sunday</td><td>NOTES:</td><td></td></tr>
<tr><td>BREAKFAST

LUNCH

DINNER

SNACK</td><td></td><td></td></tr>
</table>

Meal Planner Journal

Week of:

Monday

BREAKFAST

LUNCH

DINNER

SNACK

Tuesday

BREAKFAST

LUNCH

DINNER

SNACK

Wednesday

BREAKFAST

LUNCH

DINNER

SNACK

Thursday

BREAKFAST

LUNCH

DINNER

SNACK

Friday

BREAKFAST

LUNCH

DINNER

SNACK

Saturday

BREAKFAST

LUNCH

DINNER

SNACK

Sunday

BREAKFAST

LUNCH

DINNER

SNACK

NOTES:

Meal Planner Journal

Week of:

Monday	Tuesday	Wednesday
BREAKFAST	BREAKFAST	BREAKFAST
LUNCH	LUNCH	LUNCH
DINNER	DINNER	DINNER
SNACK	SNACK	SNACK

Thursday	Friday	Saturday
BREAKFAST	BREAKFAST	BREAKFAST
LUNCH	LUNCH	LUNCH
DINNER	DINNER	DINNER
SNACK	SNACK	SNACK

Sunday	NOTES:
BREAKFAST	
LUNCH	
DINNER	
SNACK	

WEEKLY —

Meal Planner Journal

Week of:

Monday
BREAKFAST
LUNCH
DINNER
SNACK

Tuesday
BREAKFAST
LUNCH
DINNER
SNACK

Wednesday
BREAKFAST
LUNCH
DINNER
SNACK

Thursday
BREAKFAST
LUNCH
DINNER
SNACK

Friday
BREAKFAST
LUNCH
DINNER
SNACK

Saturday
BREAKFAST
LUNCH
DINNER
SNACK

Sunday
BREAKFAST
LUNCH
DINNER
SNACK

NOTES:

Meal Planner Journal

Week of:

Monday
BREAKFAST
LUNCH
DINNER
SNACK

Tuesday
BREAKFAST
LUNCH
DINNER
SNACK

Wednesday
BREAKFAST
LUNCH
DINNER
SNACK

Thursday
BREAKFAST
LUNCH
DINNER
SNACK

Friday
BREAKFAST
LUNCH
DINNER
SNACK

Saturday
BREAKFAST
LUNCH
DINNER
SNACK

Sunday
BREAKFAST
LUNCH
DINNER
SNACK

NOTES:

WEEKLY —

Meal Planner Journal

Week of:

Monday		Tuesday		Wednesday
BREAKFAST		BREAKFAST		BREAKFAST
LUNCH		LUNCH		LUNCH
DINNER		DINNER		DINNER
SNACK		SNACK		SNACK

Thursday		Friday		Saturday
BREAKFAST		BREAKFAST		BREAKFAST
LUNCH		LUNCH		LUNCH
DINNER		DINNER		DINNER
SNACK		SNACK		SNACK

Sunday		NOTES:
BREAKFAST		
LUNCH		
DINNER		
SNACK